WHAT E

After returning from his journey through the shadowland of suffering from autoimmune illness, Dr. Guliyev brings to us an encyclopedic compendium describing the steps that led to his own cure and which he offers to others. His personal experience and training as a physician and scientist make for a compelling work that many will benefit from. The book focuses on the dependence of the immune system on digestive function and how dysbiosis, inflammation, and leaky and lazy gut can disrupt health. This volume is akin to an owner's manual for gut and immune health and a vade mecum, a handbook to consult repeatedly on the journey towards better health. Those without health issues will also benefit from learning the important steps to maintaining gut function and preventing future illness.

PHILIP PANZARELLA, MD, MPH, FACP |
CLINICAL ASSOCIATE PROFESSOR, UNIVERSITY
OF MARYLAND SCHOOL OF MEDICINE

As someone who has lived with Crohn's disease for many years, it's important to me to focus on holistic ways to support my digestive health as an adjunct to clinical treatment. Dr Anar Guliyev's book is a rich source of information on the gut microbiome, immunity, and the gut and how we might better understand the complex interplay between them all. I recommend this highly readable book to anyone wanting to benefit their gastrointestinal health.

RACHEL SAWYER | PATIENT ADVOCATE &
EDUCATOR | FOUNDER, *THE BOTTOM LINE IBD*
AND *IBD WOMEN* (UK)

Dr. Guliyev has penned a definitive book on autoimmune disorders and autoimmunity for medical professionals and the general public. He eloquently touches on the science and describes *DILL+* and the *5R+* system approach. He coined the term *Lazy Gut* to pair alongside *Leaky Gut*. Dr. Guliyev illustrates a step-by-step process for treating AI disorders and more. This book is the new blueprint and playbook for clinicians and an educational tool for the public. Anar maps out a new holistic approach to recognizing these conditions and alternative, bespoke treatment options. A must-read for any clinician treating AI diseases, holistic/integrative or allopathic.

YUSUF (JP) SALEEBY, MD CTP | FOUNDER, PRIORITY HEALTH ACADEMY & CAROLINA HOLISTIC MEDICINE | SENIOR FELLOW, FLCCC ALLIANCE | PROFESSOR OF MEDICAL ETHICS & RFXMED FOR PHA | AUTHOR

An in-depth, evidence-based exploration of the immune system, presenting it as part of a larger ecosystem. What sets this book apart is its lack of salesmanship—no gimmicks or products to buy, just clear, actionable advice using readily available resources. The author focuses on the root causes of immune dysfunction and goes beyond conventional medicine, incorporating lifestyle changes and microbiome health. I highly recommend *Autoimmunity Unlocked* to anyone seeking a science-backed approach. Whether navigating an autoimmune illness or aiming to improve overall health, this book is a must-read.

RUSLAN MAMMADOV, MD, PHD | RESEARCHER, PROJECT LEAD, DEPARTMENT OF GASTROENTEROLOGY AND HEPATOLOGY, ERASMUS MEDICAL CENTER (NETHERLANDS)

No matter if you are a patient suffering from an autoimmune disorder or somebody interested in the most up-to-date information about the close bidirectional interactions between the immune system, the gut, and its microbiome, you will find easily understandable and actionable information in Dr. Guliyev's book *Autoimmunity Unlocked*. This is one of the rare books that provides evidence-based information while calling out myths propagated in the media by self-declared experts.

EMERAN MAYER, MD | GASTROENTEROLOGIST, NEUROSCIENTIST, UCLA BRAIN-GUT-MICROBIOME EXPERT | AUTHOR, *THE MIND-GUT IMMUNE CONNECTION* | HOST, *MIND-GUT CONVERSATION*

I admire the comprehensiveness of *Autoimmunity Unlocked* — it will certainly help thousands on their journey to greater health.

TOM O'BRYAN, DC, CCN, DACBN | AUTHOR, *THE AUTOIMMUNE FIX* | PRODUCER, *BETRAYAL: THE AUTOIMMUNE DISEASE SOLUTION THEY'RE NOT TELLING YOU.*

This book stands out as an invaluable resource, taking a functional medicine and holistic approach to autoimmunity. Its clear, easy-to-understand format, complete with insightful text and helpful diagrams, makes even complex concepts accessible to those without a medical degree. Comprehensive and thoughtfully designed, it equips readers with knowledge of the factors contributing to autoimmune disorders and practical strategies (the 5R+ system of holistic healing) that can lead to meaningful recovery. I am excited to recommend this book to my clients as a trustworthy guide on their health journey.

SHARON WALT, PHD | CERTIFIED FUNCTIONAL MEDICINE HEALTH COACH | DIRECTOR, HEALTHYLIVINGWITHDRSHARON.COM

Over the decades I have taught for the Institute for Functional Medicine, I have emphasized that unless there is a compelling reason to do otherwise, one should start in the Gut. Dr. Guliyev's new book *Autoimmunity Unlocked* will take you on an extraordinary journey to the depths of why and how the gut can be the source of autoimmunity or the fountain of wellness. If you or a loved one is grappling with an autoimmune condition, this book is a must-read.

THOMAS A. SULT, MD | AUTHOR OF *JUST BE WELL: A BOOK FOR SEEKERS OF VIBRANT HEALTH.*

An exceptional read. I was impressed by the depth of coverage and sound biological rationale behind this exploration of gut health and its crucial role in immunity and disease prevention. With dietary guidance and the 5R+ framework, this book is a valuable resource for anyone seeking to improve their health.

FAYTH MILES-BUTLER, PHD | ASSOCIATE PROFESSOR, CENTER FOR NUTRITION, HEALTHY LIFESTYLES, AND DISEASE PREVENTION, LOMA LINDA UNIVERSITY

Autoimmunity Unlocked offers a groundbreaking approach to managing debilitating autoimmune conditions. This guide empowers patients with practical strategies to heal and balance their microbiome, strengthen immunity, and optimize digestive health—paving the way to improved overall well-being. It's a must-read for anyone seeking to take control of their health journey through science-backed insights and actionable steps.

SANMEET SINGH, MD | ADVANCED ENDOSCOPY, GASTROENTEROLOGY & HEPATOLOGY, DIRECTOR OF ENDOSCOPY, LUMINIS HEALTH ANNE ARUNDEL MEDICAL CENTER

Autoimmunity Unlocked masterfully bridges the gap between cutting-edge microbiome science and practical health strategies. Dr. Guliyev's integration of the latest research on gut health, immune function, and systemic wellness is both thorough and accessible. The 5R framework - Repopulate, Reduce, Repair, Reawaken, and Recondition - is a brilliantly structured, holistic approach that addresses the root causes of autoimmune conditions with precision. This book is an essential guide for anyone seeking to transform their health by unlocking the interconnected power of the microbiome, immunity, and lifestyle.

AMINE ZORGANI, PHD | FOUNDER, THE
MICROBIOME MAVERICKS | FOUNDER,
SWIPEBIOME (FRANCE)

Dr. Guliyev combines scientific knowledge with practical advice, making complex concepts accessible to readers. The numerous tables throughout the book are particularly helpful, as they guide readers in navigating their choices, making it easier to stick to the recommendations. The author's journey is inspiring and informative, offering a roadmap for anyone seeking to enhance their well-being. Filled with actionable tips, recipes, and a wealth of knowledge, this book empowers readers to take control of their health. Bring this book to your doctor so you can both work on improving your health.

ROBERT V SHIRINOV, MD, RVT, ABLS |
SURGEON, USA VEIN CLINICS

It deserves to be read by medical professionals and laypeople who sincerely want to learn more about lifestyle practices, nutritional principles, and other factors associated with better health.

NORBERT RESTREPO, PHD | PRESIDENT,
HARTLAND INSTITUTE OF HEALTH &
EDUCATION

Dr. Guliyev provides clear, well-researched, and evidence-based recommendations that address the root causes of the pain and suffering associated with autoimmune processes. His book is an excellent blueprint to follow for anyone dealing with an autoimmune condition.

MICHAEL T. MURRAY, ND | CHIEF SCIENTIFIC
ADVISOR, IHERB.COM | COAUTHOR, *A
TEXTBOOK OF NATURAL MEDICINE* AND *THE
ENCYCLOPEDIA OF NATURAL MEDICINE*

As a clinically trained specialist, I greatly appreciate the depth and clarity of this book. Dr. Guliyev has created a remarkable guide, blending well-researched, practical strategies with expert, evidence-based clinical insights offering real hope and effective solutions for those navigating autoimmune conditions.

MICHAEL ASH, DO, ND, RNT | FOUNDER,
CLINICALEDUCATION.ORG | DIRECTOR,
NUTRI-LINK (UK)

Autoimmune diseases are complex, with many causes that must be addressed. Dr. Guliyev effectively provides a comprehensive approach that is easy to understand and is highly effective.

JOSEPH E. PIZZORNO, JR., ND | PRESIDENT,
SALUGENECISTS, INC. | PRESIDENT EMERITUS,
BASTYR UNIVERSITY | EDITOR-IN-CHIEF,
*INTEGRATIVE MEDICINE: A CLINICIAN'S
JOURNAL (IMCJ)* | AUTHOR, *TOTAL WELLNESS*,
COAUTHOR, *TEXTBOOK OF NATURAL
MEDICINE*

AUTOIMMUNITY UNLOCKED

5 KEYS TO TRANSFORM MICROBIOME, IMMUNE, AND DIGESTIVE HEALTH AND RECLAIM YOUR LIFE. A 5R+ HOLISTIC GUIDE FOR RHEUMATOID ARTHRITIS, LUPUS, AND CROHN'S (ENCYCLOPEDIC EDITION)

ANAR R GULIYEV, M.D.

— INVENT & DISCOVER —

Autoimmunity Unlocked. 5 Keys to Transform Microbiome, Immune, and Digestive Health and Reclaim Your Life. A 5R+ Holistic Guide for Rheumatoid Arthritis, Lupus, and Crohn's (Encyclopedic Edition)

www.autoimmunityunlocked.org

Copyright © 2025 by Anar R Guliyev, M.D.

All rights reserved.

College Station, TX

Editors: David Stone, MS and Wendy Lord, RD.

Library of Congress Control Number: 2024925614

ISBN: 979-8-9921187-0-4 (paperback)

ISBN: 979-8-9921187-1-1 (hardcover)

ISBN: 979-8-9921187-2-8 (ebook)

ISBN: 979-8-9921187-3-5 (audiobook)

ISBN: 978-1-9870349-6-7 (B&N, paperback)

ISBN: 978-1-9870357-1-1 (B&N, hardcover)

BRIEF CONTENTS

CONTENTS

KEY 2. INFLAMMATION: REDUCE

KEY 3. LEAKY GUT: REPAIR

KEY 4. LAZY GUT: REAWAKEN

KEY 5. FACTORS BEYOND DIGESTIVE HEALTH: RECONDITION

To my parents, with heartfelt gratitude.
To Irshad, Ilyas, Amina, and Amalya, with blessings for robust health.

LEGAL DISCLAIMER

Important: Please Read Carefully Before Using This Book.

Consult a Healthcare Professional: Before following any recommendations in this book (or any other), consult your doctor or healthcare specialist.

Purpose of This Book: This book is for informational purposes only and is not intended to diagnose, treat, cure, or prevent any condition or disease. It should not be used as a substitute for consultation, diagnosis, or treatment by qualified medical practitioners.

Individual Results May Vary: The publisher and author make no guarantees about the level of success you may experience from the advice and strategies contained within. Results can differ significantly between individuals.

All efforts have been made to ensure the accuracy of the information contained in this book as of the date published. The author and the publisher expressly disclaim responsibility for any adverse effects arising from using or applying the information contained herein.

Future editions may include updates and revisions as necessary.

Author's Credentials: The author, Anar R. Guliyev, M.D., holds a medical degree. However, he is not a licensed practitioner in the United States. His professional activities are primarily focused on the fields of medtech, biotech, computer science, and health coaching.

Acceptance of Terms: By using this book, you acknowledge and agree to this disclaimer. You accept the risk that results may vary and understand that this book does not offer medical advice.

INTRODUCTION

My journey began in 1996, when, as a third-year medical student, I was diagnosed with *Rheumatoid Arthritis (RA)*, a common autoimmune disease. Within a year, my joints were so inflamed that even walking from one room to the next was a struggle. It felt as though I was bound by invisible shackles with no key in sight. Frequent eye inflammations threatened my vision and my future career. The growing array of pill bottles on my bookshelf looked like a gourmet chef's spice rack.

This daily battle with RA continued for roughly 15 years.

Fast forward to today: I am healthy, active, and pain-free. The only reason I visit a pharmacy now is for vitamins and minerals. Yes, I have been completely medication-free for over 12 years—a miracle for an RA patient—and I thank God for it. Now, I enjoy full mobility, running, and hiking regularly—activities I couldn't do in my twenties.

I want you to experience the same sense of freedom. How can you achieve this? By using the keys described in this book to unlock the health barriers that are holding you back. My miracle came in the form of understanding, a gift that can be shared with others.

This book is the result of over twenty years of research, patient coaching, and dedicated work to understand autoimmune diseases—why they start, how they progress, and what can truly make a difference—addressing the root of the problem to transform your quality of life.

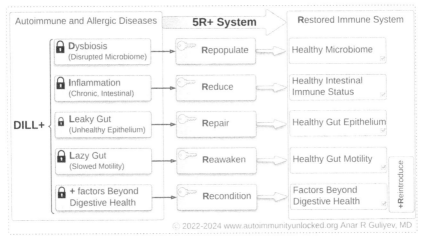

Appendix 1: Figure 1.1 - The 5 Key Components of Autoimmune Disease (DILL+)
and the 5 Elements of Holistic Healing (5R+): The Very Big Picture

I'm not offering quick fixes or typical "eat this, don't eat that" advice. Nor am I selling snake oil. Unlike many commercialized healing systems, what I provide isn't a sales pitch for any product. In fact, you can find everything you need in regular stores. If you are ready to put in the effort to improve your immune health, let me guide you.

 Your body is an ecosystem; to heal immune cells, you need to restore their entire environment.

In essence, my approach views the immune system as part of a larger **ecosystem,** made up of:

- **Immune cells**.
- The **Microbiome**—a vast and versatile community of bacteria within you.
- The **Digestive system**—home to the bulk of your microbiome and about 70% of your immune cells.

The system crystallized following my healing, when I began coaching others. Case after case, we encountered the same five factors holding the autoimmune condition in place. Once we addressed all five, it was as if invisible locks opened, allowing people to make significant progress in their healing. I call these locks **DILL+** and will explain them later.

The challenge is that all five "locks" reinforce each other, creating vicious cycles. You can't remove one without making good progress with all the rest. This requires a systematic, strategic approach, which is why many conventional and natural healing systems I know of offer only limited and temporary results.

This book is your guide to tackling all these factors simultaneously by changing your lifestyle. The **five** "**DILL+ locks**" require "**five keys**"—the five major strategies you will apply. I call this the **5R+ system**. Each strategy is complex, with multiple tactics, tips, and hints. Immune system diseases are complicated, and restoring your body's ecosystem can't be achieved with a few simple pieces of advice.

Are you reading this book because you've been diagnosed with an autoimmune disease like *Lupus* or *Rheumatoid Arthritis*? Or, do you have allergies? Maybe you picked up this book because someone you care about is struggling with an autoimmune condition, and you want to help. Whatever your reason, if you're looking to break free from the shackles of chronic inflammation and take control over your life, I understand—I've been there.

Immune system disorders come in many forms. Not only do they cause pain and inflammation, but they also make you more prone to infections and increase the risk of cancer. The limitations that accompany these conditions can be overwhelming, and all you want is to live a full, unrestricted life. I am excited to share my system with you, and I hope you will share it with others.

You'll discover how closely the microbiome is connected to more than just your immune system. Poor gut health and the microbiome affect each other as well as the immune system, increasing your chances of developing other issues like anemia, osteoporosis, obesity, diabetes, Alzheimer's, and cancer. As you read through these pages, you will see that the principles benefit everyone, whether or not they have an autoimmune disease or allergy.

Everyone's body is unique, with its own strengths, weaknesses, and challenges. I will address the most common variations based on my clinical experience, explaining how to personalize the strategies to suit your needs. Some readers might prefer to focus on the practical guidelines and skip the detailed explanations. Others will find value in understanding the "why" and "how" behind the process. This knowledge empowers you to fine-tune your approach as needed.

As a reader, you don't need any specialized knowledge or training. All explanations are simple and clear. Yet, I don't compromise on scientific accuracy, ensuring that my recommendations are fully backed by medical research.

I wrote this book to help you succeed on your healing journey. We will get straight to the point—what is broken, why it happened, and how to fix it. *Appendix 1* provides diagrams, tables, and video guides to deepen your understanding. If you're interested in further reading, you'll find references in *Appendix 2*.

As I've already said, this is not a sales pitch, and I will not commercialize anything. My goal is to help you achieve good health by *understanding* the factors that influence your immune system and *implementing* strategic lifestyle changes. Everything you need is available at the stores you visit every day. By addressing the body as a whole, true healing is often possible. You will soon see dramatic, lasting improvements in your health.

Many medical professionals believe that autoimmune diseases are incurable. Within the limits of conventional healthcare—with its reliance on medication and isolated dietary changes—they are right. Healing can only be achieved through a complete lifestyle transformation. Yes, this requires commitment and dedication, but I have seen great success in those who follow this program. Now, it's your turn.

Are you ready? Let's get started.

HOPE IN THE FACE
OF THE INCURABLE

After your initial diagnosis, you likely followed a treatment plan focused on managing your symptoms and slowing the disease progression. Life without autoimmune disease was not in the cards.

Yet, I'm here to tell you that regaining health after a severe autoimmune condition is often possible. It may seem like a bold statement, but it is supported by my personal experience, as well as the many people who have subsequently followed this program and experienced healing. You don't have to accept your condition as inevitable—you have the power to live the active life you want, free from chronic inflammation.

So, are autoimmune diseases incurable or not? The short answer is: yes. Within the limitations of the conventional healthcare system, autoimmune diseases are typically incurable. Treatments mainly aim to manage the disease and reduce symptoms.

The long answer, though, is much more encouraging. By taking a holistic approach—making lifestyle changes and strategically targeting multiple aspects of your body—you can overhaul your bacterial landscape to transform your immune system and significantly improve your health. In many cases, I've even witnessed complete cures. But before we delve into how you can achieve this, let's discuss why conventional medicine is limited.

Conventional healthcare relies on methods that are *scalable, repro-*

ducible, and *feasible.* Doctors need to deliver consistent results and help as many patients as possible with restricted time and resources. Any highly personalized strategies that depend heavily on the patient's hard work and lifestyle changes over many years just cannot be accommodated.

Today, most medical treatments involve taking medications to correct what's wrong by influencing the body's chemical reactions. This approach gets the job done quickly, enabling doctors to treat more patients within an overburdened healthcare system.

Sometimes, *adding* something new can be efficient, but it is not always a solution. Often, you will see better results by *subtracting* something—like an unhealthy food or habit—or making fundamental lifestyle *changes.* The problem is, this requires effort, self-discipline, and dedication. Results take time, and many people lose interest when they don't see immediate improvements. Your doctor simply doesn't have the time to guide you through an intensive transformation. Instead, the medication cycle continues, leaving people with autoimmune diseases frustrated and searching for better answers. Side effects are common. No matter how small they are, they build up over time, creating new problems and further limiting the effectiveness of drugs in managing chronic diseases.

> A placebo is a treatment that has no real medical benefit but can sometimes improve a person's condition due to the power of belief.

Now, let's discuss why natural treatments often fall short. Many natural healing plans boil down to "eat this; it will help." Basically, instead of adding a pharmacy-bought product, you add one bought at a supermarket or, worse, an overpriced supplement marketed online by an enterprising healing guru.

These products might be helpful, and they are generally safe—nobody wants to be sued. They are also available without a prescription because their effects are usually weak. Such supplements cannot cure complex illnesses on their own. Sometimes, we even come across websites selling 'remedies' that don't make any scientific sense. If they work for someone, it's usually due to the *placebo effect.*

Most self-proclaimed healers are just selling placebos with a hefty markup.

To avoid the placebo-market traps, always scrutinize the scientific explanation of **how** something works. Also, check if the claims are supported by independent scientific publications in reputable journals.

 If a treatment can't be scientifically explained, it's either a miracle or a scam. If you have to pay for it, it's probably the latter.

Because "eat this" methods don't solve the problem, many people with autoimmune disorders keep switching from one medication to another—following their doctor's advice—while chasing the latest "miracle cures" they find online. People often resist making fundamental lifestyle changes. Instead, they search for a magic pill (or a magic plant, for

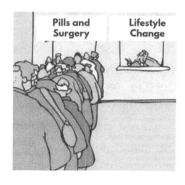

those who prefer natural healing) that promises a miracle cure without much effort. This doesn't work, and the struggle to find a genuine solution continues.

 No miracle food or supplement can replace the need for a lifestyle change.

Recovering from an autoimmune disease is complex. The immune system is interconnected with various other aspects of your body—the *microbiome*, the digestive system, hormones, sleep patterns, physical activity, and more. Targeting one or two of these processes at a time is not enough. You need to address many factors at once to make real progress. A common mistake is to treat the most obvious issues while ignoring others. These unchanged aspects continually pull you back towards the disease as if being tied to it by rubber bands.

The human microbiome is a community of
trillions of bacteria and other microorganisms
living within and on the surface of our body.
These living microorganisms play a significant
role in health and disease, influencing your
metabolism, immune system, and other
functions. While specialists sometimes
differentiate between the microbiota (the
microorganisms) and the microbiome (the
microorganisms along with their genes), for
simplicity, we will use these terms
interchangeably in this book.

Doctors understand these connections and may address some of them, but it's not practical for them to manage everything. They don't have the time required to guide each patient through a significant lifestyle revamp. This requires self-discipline and a commitment from you that doctors can't enforce. It is more efficient for them to focus on strategies that work best for most of their patients. This means that, despite all the supporting research, addressing the root causes of many complex illnesses in modern healthcare settings is not feasible.

Adding to the challenge, researchers have only relatively recently started unraveling the links between the immune system and the microbiome. It is a complex dynamic ecosystem, with natural selection, competition, survival of the fittest, and population changes. You cannot restructure something as intricate as an *ecological community* with medication or isolated dietary changes.

An ecosystem is a community of living
organisms, such as plants, animals, and
microbes, that interact with each other and
their physical environment within a specific
area.

Your body is not a collection of separate systems, and your treatment plan should reflect that. The holistic approach in this book is based on years of experience and systematically targets several fundamental areas that are interconnected with the immune system. If you have an autoimmune disease, problems in these areas support the condition. I call them the **5 "DILL+" locks**. Corresponding to these locks are the **5 "R" keys**—the core strategies of our system that restore the foundational pillars. Finally, there is a "Reintroduce" step, where you can bring back many of the foods you had to exclude during the strict elimination diet phase. This is why it is called the **5R+ System**. It is not only about food; each key incorporates many other essential factors. This book has 5 sections, each focusing on a specific lock-and-key pair.

We'll talk a lot about digestive health, which needs serious repair in many people. For example, you might have heard of **Leaky Gut** syndrome, which results from an unhealthy gut lining (*epithelium*). Fewer people know about what I call **Lazy Gut**—a condition of poor *gut motility* (movement). Both of these conditions affect your immune health. We will also cover issues like hidden **intestinal Inflammation**, oral health, unhealthy stomach juices and bile, and more. While diet and digestive health are crucial, they are only part of the puzzle. There are other factors beyond the digestive system—the "+" in the **DILL+** locks mentioned earlier. We'll explore these in the final section of the book.

And, of course, we will explore the **Microbiome** in detail. We will work on improving it in two ways—its **Distribution** and its **Composition**. Fixing the *distribution* will address problems such as **IBS (Irritable Bowel Syndrome)** and **SIBO (Small Intestinal Bacterial Overgrowth)**, both of which are often linked to autoimmune diseases. Restoring the *composition* will strengthen your entire internal ecosystem, making it more stable and resilient against occasional diet deviations and infections. It also ensures more robust immunity.

When I was a medical student, the scientific community knew very little about the human microbiome. Even today, we are only just beginning to grasp how it impacts our health. The concept of "Leaky Gut" was also unknown. By God's grace, in the early 2000s, I began learning how the immune system is connected to the vast world of our body's bacteria and internal ecosystem factors, all of which shape its function. The good news is that these elements can be modified to potentially restore a healthy microbiome and immune system. The holistic approach goes beyond diet. Indeed, much of it is about food, but we will also discuss seemingly unrelated factors like hormones, the micro-climate in your home, mold exposure, abdominal muscle strength, and even snoring. This system took many years of research, experimenta-tion, and learning from patients I had the privilege to coach. I am grateful for the deeper understanding I have gained, and I am excited to share it with you.

The system requires significant lifestyle changes—some temporary, some permanent. Each of the 5R+ keys is complex and involves multiple tactics. By understanding how everything is connected—the what, why, and how things are happening—you'll be better motivated and equipped to identify and handle any setbacks. These locks, keys, and tactics are illustrated in a free mind map, available for download in *Bonus 1*.

Changing a habit is difficult, but as the saying goes, "The definition of insanity is doing the same thing over and over and expecting different results." It's time to stop searching for a miracle cure. Instead, you will find health through a consistent strategy that requires dedica-tion and self-discipline to rebuild your health on multiple fronts.

Yes, the immune system is complex. That's why this book is lengthy. The good news is that this process is inexpensive. Unlike some other books you may have read, I am not trying to sell you anything! All you need is determination. You'll change many of your habits; your diet and lifestyle will differ significantly from your friends. And then comes the great news. Your overall health—not just your immune system—will improve dramatically.

You may have heard the phrase, "What got you here won't get you there." Let's start by exploring how to get "*there*". If you haven't already done so, download the complete mind map from *Bonus 1*. It's free, and I encourage you to share it with others who might benefit. The map might look overwhelming at first, but don't worry—you'll become familiar with it as we go through each key and tactic step by step. It is the map of your healing journey; this book is your guide. A journey of a thousand miles begins with a single step, and you just took that step by opening this book. In fact, you've already read 3% of it!

———

Important: Always consult a physician if you notice any unusual or uncomfortable symptoms.

- Your condition should improve, not worsen.
- The only discomfort you should experience is hunger during water fasting.
- If you have diabetes or other medical conditions, fasting may not be appropriate. Consult your doctor first.
- If something goes wrong or simply does not feel right, consult your doctor.
- Avoid any foods that cause intolerance or allergic reactions, even if they are on the recommended foods list; focus on those you tolerate well. As you restore your immune system, you may become allergy-free and can add them back later under your doctor's guidance.
- Do not reduce or discontinue any medication without talking to your doctor first.

The goal is to help you build a foundation where medication becomes unnecessary. This process will take time. As you progress, your doctor will notice improvements and may consider changes in your treatment plan.

 Consult your doctor before following the recommendations in this book or any other.

IMMUNE SYSTEM — THE GOOD, THE BAD, AND THE UGLY

➕ BONUS 1.
COMPLETE MIND
MAP OF 5R+ KEYS AND TACTICS

Download the full-color, comprehensive mind map of All 5R+ Keys and Tactics: https://bonus.autoimmunityunlocked.org/

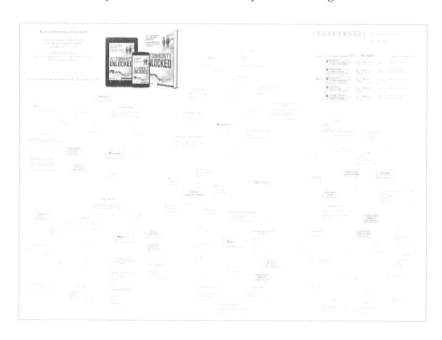

THE UGLY: AN AILING IMMUNE SYSTEM

DISEASES RELATED TO IMMUNE SYSTEM DISORDERS

Let's begin with the ugly side of autoimmune disease, which is just one kind of immune system dysfunction. Most patients suffer from one dominant condition, but it is seldom their only concern—related issues often follow. Immune system problems typically fall into one of these categories:

- Autoimmune diseases (Lupus, Rheumatoid Arthritis, Hashimoto Thyroiditis, etc.)
- Allergies
- Susceptibility to infections
- Increased risk of certain cancers

Though this book focuses mainly on autoimmune diseases, the method outlined for restoring the immune system can help with all of these conditions.

THE IMMUNE SYSTEM AND CANCER — A HIDDEN LINK
It is obvious that chronic inflammation exhausts the immune cells,

leading to a greater risk of infections. The link between the immune system and cancer, however, needs more clarification.

Cell mutations occur regularly in our bodies. A healthy immune system recognizes and destroys these mutated cells early. However, a compromised immune system is less efficient, missing the target and letting some cells escape and spread. This is an oversimplified explanation—there are various ways cancer hides from the immune system, which are beyond the scope of this book.

Fortunately, advancements in *immunotherapy* in oncology are showing great promise. This link between the immune system and cancer only solidifies my belief that the principles outlined in this book can greatly benefit those living with tumors and can be used as a preventative tool for those who want to reduce their risk significantly.

> Lymphocytes are a type of white blood cell, a large family of immune cells with two main classes: T-lymphocytes control your body's immune response and directly attack and kill infected and tumor cells. B-lymphocytes produce antibodies—proteins that target viruses, bacteria, and toxins.

We know there is a strong link between cancer and chronic inflammation, and people with an autoimmune disease are more likely to develop malignancies. For example, rheumatoid arthritis (RA) patients have a higher risk of being diagnosed with lymphomas. You can see why, then, it is crucial to work on restoring a healthy immune system. True healing only begins when you address the root cause instead of masking your symptoms with immunosuppressants.

AUTOIMMUNE DISEASES — A MODERN EPIDEMIC

Autoimmune diseases are not only becoming more common, but they are also affecting younger people. Before the mid-20th century, cases of autoimmune disorders were relatively rare. Today, in the United States, about 8% of the population is officially diagnosed with an autoimmune disease, a rate higher than that of heart disease or cancer. And that doesn't account for undiagnosed cases. When including mild and undiagnosed cases, the number is estimated to be as high as 16-22%. This means that at least one in five women and one in seven men are living with an autoimmune disorder.

There are many contributing factors. Genetics is one of them, but scientists are also unraveling the strong connection between the microbiome and immune health.

In this book, we take a holistic approach to restoring your microbial community and offer tactics to improve other areas affecting immune function. Since 70% of the immune system is located in the gut, many of our strategies target the gut microbiome and digestive health. They may require significant adjustments to your routine, but they can substantially improve your overall health. Considering roughly 20% of the population has some form of food intolerance, it is clear that some diet and lifestyle changes are necessary.

See also:

• Appendix 1 ➤ Figures 2.1, 2.2, 2.3, 2.4

IMMUNE ILLNESS ON THE RISE

Historical data shows that food allergies and intolerances were rare up until the mid-20th century. Since the 1950s, however, rates of multiple sclerosis, Crohn's disease, type 1 diabetes, and asthma have soared by over 300%. I believe these trends are linked to changes in our microbiome, driven by modern lifestyle choices. In fact, the microbiome is the only human organ that has significantly changed over the past century, and it is closely linked to the immune system.

The impact of lifestyle becomes more apparent when we compare the prevalence of autoimmune diseases between Western nations and other countries. For instance, *ulcerative colitis*, a form of *inflammatory bowel disease (IBD)*, is more than twice as prevalent in Western Europe than it is in Eastern Europe (6.5 vs. 3.1 per 100,000 people). Similarly, in Turkey, the incidence of allergies among teenagers is 20 times lower than in Western Europe (4.2% in Germany vs. 0.15% in Turkey.) Unfortunately, as Westernized diets and lifestyles spread globally, we are seeing a rise in these conditions worldwide.

See also:

• Appendix 1 ➣ Figure 2.1, 2.2

WHEN THE BODY ATTACKS ITSELF

Autoimmune disease occurs when the immune system mistakenly attacks the body's own healthy cells—unable to distinguish them from foreign invaders. Depending on which organs and tissues are targeted, this can lead to one of the multitude of autoimmune diseases we now know. Here are some of the most common:

- Addison's Disease
- Celiac Disease (Gluten-Sensitive Enteropathy)
- Dermatomyositis
- Grave's Disease
- Hashimoto Thyroiditis
- Inflammatory Bowel Disease (IBD) (Crohn's Disease, Ulcerative Colitis, etc.)
- Multiple Sclerosis
- Myasthenia Gravis
- Pernicious Anemia
- Reactive Arthritis
- Rheumatoid Arthritis (RA)
- Sjögren Syndrome
- Systemic Lupus Erythematosus
- Type I Diabetes

According to the American Autoimmune Related Diseases Association (AARDA), there are over 150 recognized autoimmune diseases. A full list is available in *Appendix 1*. Although each disease requires specific treatments (as your doctor would have explained), the basic approach to restoring a healthy immune system through changing its ecosystem remains the same.

See also:

• Appendix 1 ➣ Figure 2.3, 2.4

THE BAD: WHY CONVENTIONAL TREATMENTS ARE LIMITED

The standard approach to treating autoimmune diseases is to suppress the immune system. But what happens when this strategy reaches its limit? Routinely increasing the dosage of immunosuppressants is not a sustainable solution—you can't shut down your immune system entirely. Also, prolonged use of these medications increases the risk of side effects. Since the drugs suppress proliferating cells, patients are likely to develop anemia, fertility problems, ulcers (especially with the use of NSAIDs), and more. Additionally, a weakened immune system makes you more vulnerable to cancer and infections, as mentioned previously.

> The epithelium is a thin layer of cells covering body surfaces that acts as a protective barrier. The gut epithelium lines the inside of the digestive tract. It prevents harmful substances from entering the body while allowing the absorption of nutrients. It is an essential component of the digestive system and is crucial in maintaining overall health and wellness.

One critical issue is how these medications negatively affect the regeneration of the *intestinal epithelium*. The natural function of gut bacteria—an essential part of the immune system—is also disrupted, worsening leaky gut and chronic inflammation and, in some cases, causing ulcers.

> The main classes of drugs used to suppress the immune system in autoimmune diseases include: Nonsteroidal anti-inflammatory drugs (NSAIDs), Corticosteroids (hormonal drugs), Disease-modifying antirheumatic drugs (DMARDs).

You've probably read about your medication's side effects; maybe you've even experienced some. I remember being prescribed *Methotrexate, Hydroxychloroquine, Diclofenac, Meloxicam,* etc, when I was only 20 years old, fearing what my forties would bring. Thankfully, with God's help, I found a better way, and I've been medication-free for over 12 years.

Important: Do not change or stop any prescribed medications without consulting your doctor. The system in this book will gradually help rebuild your immune health and reduce disease activity. As your health improves, your doctor may consider reducing or discontinuing medication based on clinical and laboratory results. Collaboration with your doctor is critical; always be open about your plans. If needed, seek a second opinion from another doctor. This process is gradual—it may take months or even years. (It took me many years. However, being equipped with the 5R+ System roadmap, your journey should be faster.) The longer you have been sick, the longer it may take you to return to health, so be patient.

WHY THE AUTOIMMUNE PROTOCOL (AIP), ELIMINATION DIETS, AND PROBIOTIC SUPPLEMENTS ARE SHORT-TERM SOLUTIONS

Many people try natural healing methods but often see inconsistent and temporary improvements. The disease may "hibernate"—go into remission—only to "reawaken" when triggered by stress, an infection, or small changes to your diet. Most naturopathic approaches address only a few aspects of a multi-faceted problem—typically the most obvious ones, such as inflammation. When isolated, they yield unreliable results. What's truly needed is a strategic combination of multiple techniques working synergistically to attack the problem from every angle.

The most common naturopathic method is the Autoimmune Protocol diet (AIP). It works to a degree because it excludes foods known to cause sensitivities. However, it only addresses part of the intestinal ecosystem. Removing some of what you eat is not enough to eliminate inflammation when you are dealing with a disrupted microbiome, compromised epithelium, and poor *motility*. In fact, your body may start reacting to even more foods over time, and avoiding all of them is impossible. Unfortunately, this happens to many patients.

> Gastrointestinal (GI) Motility refers to the muscle movements that help pass food through the digestive tract. At the same time, they ensure the absorption of essential nutrients, the removal of by-products and toxins, and the regulation of the colonization of the gut microbiome. The synchronized contraction of these muscles is called peristalsis.

In *Key 2, Inflammation: Reduce*, we'll explore why simply cutting out foods (as in the AIP) is not a long-term solution for reducing inflammation. Although the basic principles of the AIP are sound, they need to be part of a broader strategy for lasting results. That's why, in one of our key strategies, the AIP is combined with additional tactics to tackle inflammation effectively.

Probiotics are another useful tool for restoring your microbiome. Still, they won't work unless you address other factors like digestive juices, bile, inflammation, and motility as well. In some cases, like *small intestinal bacterial overgrowth (SIBO)*, taking pre- and probiotics can even be harmful if these other issues aren't resolved first. Probiotics are one of the tactics we use in *Key 1: Microbiome: Repopulate*. We'll cover how to include these in your food and maximize their efficacy. In addition, I share delicious recipes of naturally fermented foods. Check them out in *Bonus 2*.

Most advice focuses only on diet, eliminating foods that trigger immune responses. They don't address the root cause of the problem, so the effects are temporary and limited. Meanwhile, immunosuppressive medications have detrimental side effects. What, then, is the answer?

We need to treat the **whole ecosystem** by addressing these three elements **simultaneously**:

- Immune system
- Digestive health
- Microbiome

In the next chapter, we will paint the big picture of this holistic approach.

THE GOOD: THE HOLISTIC WAY TO RESTORE IMMUNE HEALTH

IMMUNE CELLS IN YOUR BODY'S ECOSYSTEM

An *ecosystem* is the entire environment and its community—the landscape, climate, plants, and animals. If one thing changes, the rest changes, too. Think of a forest: if you cut down trees, different animals will inhabit the space. Remove the rabbits, and soon the foxes disappear. Add more rain, and the vegetation changes, causing some animals to become extinct while others thrive. I've oversimplified the concept, but you get the idea.

The same is true of your body—it is an ecosystem, and your immune system is an important part of it. Roughly 2 trillion lymphocytes—the immune cells that keep you healthy—coexist with about 39 trillion bacteria of your microbiome. They affect and interact with each other. Together, they rely on the "landscape and climate"—the work of all other organs and tissues and the type and quality of food you feed them. With this in mind, autoimmune disease is not your immune system attacking your body's cells without reason; it is a problem *in* and *of* the ecosystem. So, to overcome autoimmune disorders, you must restore the entire system.

As mentioned earlier, the three main areas to address in the body's ecosystem are: digestive health, the microbiota, and the immune system. The Keys 1 through 4 focus on repairing these central pillars.

Other factors influence the ecosystem as well, which we'll cover in *Key 5. Factors Beyond Digestive Health: Recondition.*

THE FIVE PILLARS OF A HEALTHY IMMUNE SYSTEM

One of the most important parts of the digestive system is its *epithelium*. Besides its digestive function, it plays a crucial role in maintaining the health and stability of the microbiome. The combination of an intact gut lining, healthy intestinal walls, effective digestion, and gut motility creates a stable environment for your immune system. In this balanced ecosystem, your microbiome and your immune cells can live together in harmony.

With a healthy gut as the foundation, I consider the five main factors for a healthy immune system to be:

- Healthy microbiome
- Healthy immune conditions in the intestine (no chronic inflammation)
- Healthy gut epithelium
- Healthy gut motility
- + Factors beyond digestive health

These components influence and support each other, as shown in Figure 2.5. Like an arch, all the bricks need to be in place for the structure to stay up. Also like an arch, once that happens, it's a powerful structure that can support other things.

Scientists have recently begun to see the *microbiome* as a unique organ in the human body. It is a community of microorganisms that continually challenge and compete with your immune cells, affecting how they function. Gut bacteria also synthesize substances we need for a healthy gut epithelium and proper gut motility.

A healthy *epithelium* is the barrier separating the outside of your body from your internal tissues. It prevents large molecules from entering your bloodstream and contacting your immune cells. The epithelial cells also secrete substances that support the microbiome's normal functioning.

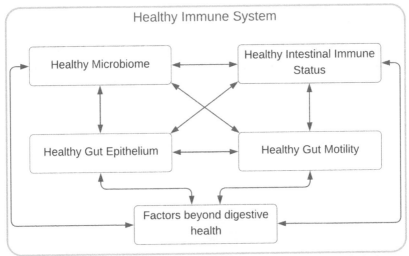

Appendix 1: Figure 2.5 - Healthy immune system factors supporting each other

Effective *motility*, the ability to move food and waste efficiently through the digestive system, is also essential. It prevents the buildup of harmful bacteria and toxins, supporting a healthy microbiome and gut lining.

We'll go into more detail about each of these aspects later.

Almost 70% of your immune system is located in the intestinal wall. Around 80% of your plasma cells are also found here. Therefore, the *immune status* of your gut defines the immune health of your entire body.

The activity level of the immune cells in the gut should be "just right"—busy but not overworked, combined with periods of relative rest and restoration. This balance of stress and rest is essential for every organ in your body. Just as your heart, muscles, and brain need time to recover after exertion, so does your immune system and gut epithelium. We'll cover more about this balancing act later.

See also:
- Appendix 1 ➢ Figure 2.5

DILL+: LOCKS AND VICIOUS CYCLES

Just as all the parts of a robust immune system support each other, so the system can collapse when something goes wrong. A problem in one area can cause a chain reaction, leading to multiple issues. Instead of a collection of *healthy* factors, you end up with a group of harmful ones that feed into each other, creating vicious cycles.

The main factors in this breakdown are:

- Dysbiosis (Disrupted microbiota)
- Intestinal Inflammation (often subclinical, without symptoms)
- Leaky Gut (Unhealthy gut epithelium)
- Lazy Gut (Impaired motility)
- + Other Factors (Beyond the digestive system)

> Dysbiosis is an imbalance in the microbial community (microbiome), where healthy bacteria are outnumbered by harmful ones, or the distribution of the bacteria shifts in an unhealthy way. Dysbiosis is most commonly reported as a medical condition in the gut microbiome.

I call the four main pathological factors **DILL**. The + (plus) refers to the additional minor factors unrelated to the digestive system. Together, these are the five locks you need to "open" to resolve your autoimmune disease.

The DILL+ system views the main components of disease as five "locks" that, when opened, free you from the "shackles" of the condition. If you have arthritis, it's easy to imagine autoimmune sickness as restraints holding you captive. I remember my inflamed joints from 20 years ago and how difficult it was to simply walk from room to room. It truly felt like being locked up.

Your microbiota—whether healthy or unhealthy—largely determine the state of your immune system. Harmful bacteria trigger immune responses, gradually changing your body's defense mechanisms, much like a chronic infection leads to ongoing inflammation. This relationship between the microbiome and immune cells is a two-way street; when one changes, so does the other. Just as animals in an ecosystem rely on each other for their survival needs, so do the microbiota and the immune system—their health and function are interdependent. We will discuss this and more in *Key 1. Dysbiosis: Repopulate.*

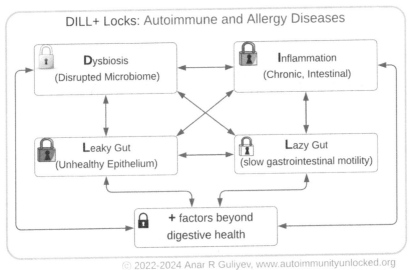

Appendix 1: Figure 2.6 - Sick immune system factors: DILL+ "locks"

As previously mentioned, most of the immune system resides in the gut, usually making digestive problems the primary concern. That's why 80% of the DILL+ system concentrates on food and digestive health. An exhausted immune system cannot effectively fight infections, allowing them to become long-term health issues. The result is chronic inflammation, which wears out the immune system, gut epithelium, and intestinal nerve cells, further slowing down motility. Most people with autoimmune diseases have a degree of symptomless, weak, but lingering inflammation in the digestive system. This creates a vicious cycle: a chronically fatigued immune system leads to impaired function, which results in continuous damage. We will cover this further in *Key 2. Inflammation: Reduce.*

Most Important Vicious Cycles of DILL+

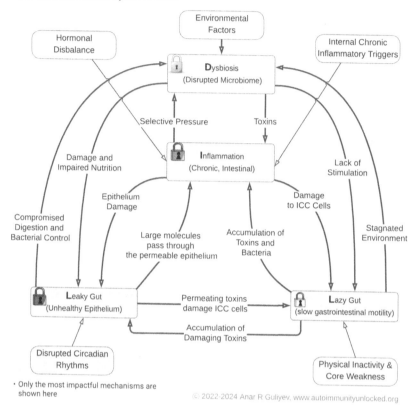

Appendix 1: Figure 2.7 - Vicious cycles of DILL+

Increased gut permeability—often called *Leaky Gut*—together with lesions on the epithelium allows incompletely digested food molecules to be absorbed. This wreaks havoc on your immune system, especially as these conditions can go unnoticed for years. Such close contact between immune cells and undigested particles triggers an abnormal immune response, leading to food sensitivities and ongoing inflammation. With increased permeability, chronic gut inflammation becomes an issue that can progress to the rest of the immune system. In addition, a damaged epithelium cannot control the digestive process well nor function as an effective barrier. Together, these factors contribute to adverse changes in the microbiome, leading to further epithelial damage. Once again, we are back to the vicious cycle of inflammation, dysbiosis, and slowed motility. We will talk about this in *Key 3. Leaky Gut: Repair.*

An inflamed gut struggles to move its contents effectively, leading to destructive stagnation. Your gut always contains some toxins—by-products of food digestion and microbial activity. An unhealthy microbiome means even more toxins. That's why active motility is vital. Slower movement causes food, toxins, and harmful bacteria to stay in the gut longer, worsening the problems. Certain bacteria grow excessively in areas they don't belong. The prolonged contact of toxins with the gut lining and immune cells triggers more irritation and inflammation. These effects further disrupt microbial populations, fueling the vicious cycle of inflammation, bacterial overgrowth, and continued damage. We'll discuss this in *Key 4. Lazy Gut: Reawaken.*

You can see how each of the DILL+ parts affects the others. One defective component impacts the rest, creating a cycle of problems.

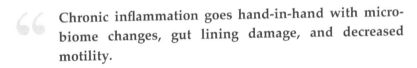

> **Chronic inflammation goes hand-in-hand with microbiome changes, gut lining damage, and decreased motility.**

That is why fixing just one issue won't work—you must address them all at the same time. This holistic approach is usually missing in various healing systems. True healing requires a comprehensive strategy; there is no single miracle food you can eat or avoid to solve everything.

See also:
• Appendix 1 ➤ Figure 2.6, 2.7

DANGERS BENEATH THE SURFACE

You might live with these conditions for years without noticeable symptoms. It's like a car with a minor oil or transmission leak—it runs fine for a while, so you don't worry about repairs. But over time, major components wear out, and one day, your car won't start. Similarly, this is how many people develop autoimmune diseases as they age. The underlying issues go unnoticed for years until something finally breaks.

That's why I recommend this system even for generally healthy people. The 5R+ principles are not a medication to take only when sick; they are a way to restore and maintain a healthy body, with a focus on immunity, the microbiome, and digestive health.

5R+: UNDERSTANDING THE HEALING STRATEGY

We've discussed what the DILL+ 'locks' are, but how do you unlock them? This book gives you the 'keys' to address each lock through the 5R+ method. See Appendix 1, Table 2.8, for how the key strategies match the problems.

Locks (DILL+)	Keys (5R+)
Dysbiosis	Repopulate the microbiome with healthy bacteria
Inflammation	Reduce inflammation
Leaky gut	Repair the intestinal epithelium
Lazy gut	Reawaken intestinal motility
+ Other pathological factors	Recondition factors beyond the digestive system
	As Your Healing Progresses:
	+ Reintroduce (gradually) healthy foods removed during the active healing phase
	These steps lead to:
	Restored immune system

Appendix 1: Figure 2.8 - DILL+ "locks" and corresponding 5R+ "keys"

All of this should be done simultaneously, not one step at a time.

Because all DILL+ factors are interconnected, you cannot change one without changing the others.

Many natural healing systems don't work because they target only part of the ecosystem—it's like changing the animals in a habitat without altering the plants or climate. The ecosystem always reverts to its previous state.

See also:
- Appendix 1 ➢ Table 2.8

5R+ IN A NUTSHELL

Throughout this process, we will work to restore your microbiome and immune system concurrently. These are the factors we'll address:

- **Key 1. Dysbiosis: Repopulate the Microbiome.** This involves improving two key aspects: the *composition* of bacterial species and the *distribution* of their populations throughout the digestive system.
- **Key 2. Inflammation: Reduce Inflammatory Processes in the Intestine.** By eliminating the chronic load on gut immune tissue, we allow it to restore normal function and structure.
- **Key 3. Leaky Gut: Repair Leaky Gut and Unhealthy Gut Epithelium.** Increased permeability, or "leakiness," is just one of many issues with an unhealthy gut lining that we must address.
- **Key 4. Lazy Gut: Reawaken Active Motility.** This focuses on promoting healthy muscle and nerve function in the digestive system to ensure efficient movement, removal of toxins, and maintenance of a healthy environment.
- **Key 5. Factors Beyond the? Digestive System: Recondition.** We address multiple factors, including environmental conditions, hormones, physical exercise, sleep and circadian rhythms, hydrotherapy, and oral health.

Each key strategy involves various tactics; some will overlap as they are relevant to several keys. Therefore, we'll explain certain tactics thoroughly in one section and refer to them again in another. This ensures you understand the *why* and *how* of each aspect before moving on to the practical *what*: to-do list. In my coaching, I have found that people heal more effectively when they understand how things work, building a new lifestyle rather than just following a list of rules. When you understand what is going on "under the hood," it becomes easier to make the necessary changes.

The exciting part is that once you have repaired all these factors, you can reintroduce some foods you had to cut out during the active healing process (like nuts, in my case). Plus, a healthy microbiome is more forgiving, allowing for the occasional cheat day.

This system requires time and discipline, although nothing extreme or overwhelming. It's about adopting an unusual healthy lifestyle. Best of all, unlike many other systems, you don't need to buy any expensive products. This is not a commercial system—I am not selling anything!

KEY 1. DYSBIOSIS: REPOPULATE THE MICROBIOME

The first key addresses the challenge of *dysbiosis*—an imbalance in your microbial community. This is the heart of the 5R+ system, demanding a detailed explanation that fills almost half the pages in this book. While Key 1 is central to restoring immune health, true healing only occurs when all the keys are addressed simultaneously.

Your body is an extraordinary machine. Each part—from your immune cells and resident bacteria to every one of your organs and tissues—is intricately connected. These cells and microbes don't just share a space; they influence and depend on each other. Changing one element invariably impacts the rest, a concept particularly true in something as extensive as the microbiome. This interdependence is precisely why the 5R+ system's other keys focus on the microbiota's habitat—the digestive system and beyond. That's also why this first key, *Repopulating the Microbiome*, is a fundamental element of our autoimmune solution. By repopulating your microbiota with beneficial bacteria, you enhance the functioning of your entire internal ecosystem.

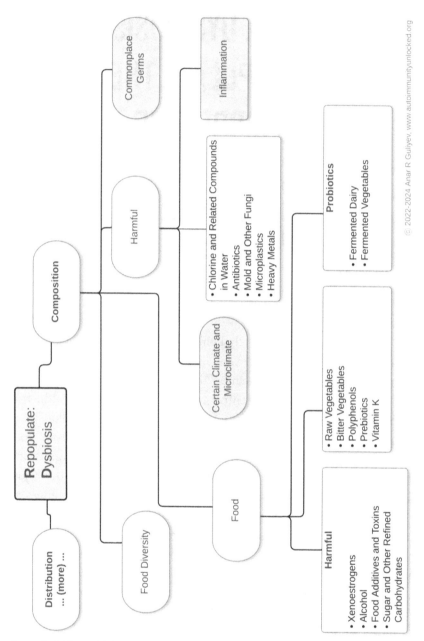

Appendix 1: Figure 3.0.1. Key 1 Tactics. Repopulate the Microbiome. Download the full-color, comprehensive mind map of All 5R+ Keys and Tactics at Bonus 1 https://bonus.autoimmunityunlocked.org/

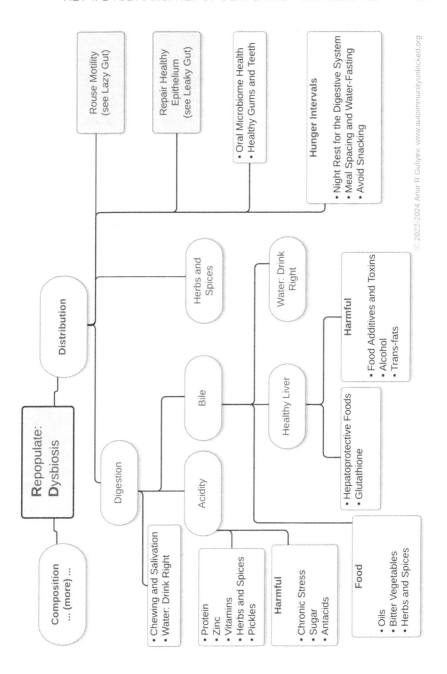

Human Microbiome
By the Numbers

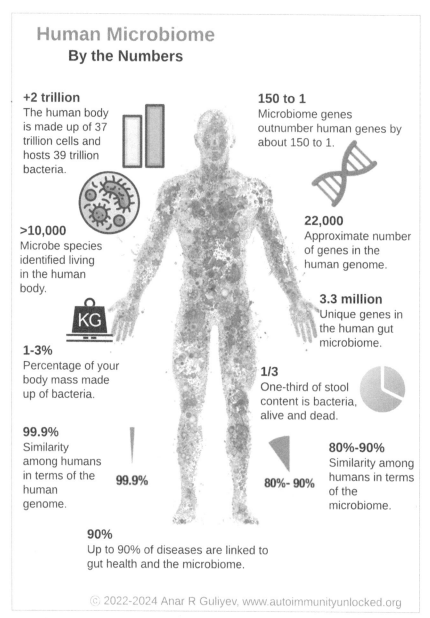

+2 trillion
The human body is made up of 37 trillion cells and hosts 39 trillion bacteria.

>10,000
Microbe species identified living in the human body.

1-3%
Percentage of your body mass made up of bacteria.

99.9%
Similarity among humans in terms of the human genome.

99.9%

90%
Up to 90% of diseases are linked to gut health and the microbiome.

150 to 1
Microbiome genes outnumber human genes by about 150 to 1.

22,000
Approximate number of genes in the human genome.

3.3 million
Unique genes in the human gut microbiome.

1/3
One-third of stool content is bacteria, alive and dead.

80%- 90%

80%-90%
Similarity among humans in terms of the microbiome.

Appendix 1: Figure 3.1. Human Microbiome by the Numbers

THE LAST DISCOVERED ORGAN THAT RESHAPES OUR UNDERSTANDING OF HEALTH

MICROBIAL FORCES WITHIN US

Did you know that the bacteria in your body outnumbers your own cells? Astonishingly, your body, composed of around 37 trillion human cells, hosts roughly 39 trillion microbes. Since they are much smaller than human cells, though, bacteria only account for about 1-3% of your body mass. Most of them are found in the gut, with both living and dead microorganisms accounting for a third of the material in your stools.

Recent studies have revealed that the gut microbiota influence virtually every organ in the body. Their effects intricately weave through various body systems, such as metabolism, digestion, hormonal balance, and mental health. There is even a link between the bacteria in your gut and your brain, referred to as the "*gut-brain axis.*" Yet, most notable is the relationship between the microbiome and the immune system.

These connections become even more fascinating when considering genetics and its role in autoimmune diseases and allergies. The human genome, your biological blueprint, consists of around 20,000 genes. In contrast, the average human microbiome is believed to contain over 3 million genes. That means less than 1% of the genes in your body's

DNA are human! While you can't alter the DNA you were born with, you *can* change the genetic composition of your bacteria.

See also:

• Appendix 1 ➤ Figure 3.1

A BUSY, ADAPTABLE ORGAN

The microbiome is viewed as either an organ or, more correctly, an organ system with multiple functions. In other words, an unhealthy microbiota is a systemic issue. Fortunately, it has a unique quality. Most organs can't alter their cells and genes. Your skin and muscles can regenerate to a certain extent, but the brain, heart, and joints have very limited regenerative capacity. The microbiota is unique—it has the remarkable ability to completely reinvent itself by repopulating its bacteria. This adaptability allows it to fluctuate between healthy and unhealthy states, primarily influenced by your lifestyle choices, which can harm or repair it.

> An ecological niche is a species' "address" within the habitat or ecosystem, covering all aspects such as location, food, available resources, and how it interacts with other organisms. It refers to where a species fits in its environment and what it does in the ecological community.

Since bacteria safeguard their *ecological niches* and prevent the entry of unwanted invaders, a healthy microbiome is a natural defense against harmful *pathogenic bacteria*. Yet, its contributions to our health are far greater than mere defense. The microbiome is also involved in:

• Digestion.
• Preventing infections and growth of pathogenic bacteria.
• Repairing the intestinal lining.
• Generating energy for the gut epithelium.
• Managing inflammation.
• Maintaining immune health.

- Vitamin production, including vitamin B_{12} and 50% of our vitamin K requirements.

We'll explore more of these functions in later sections.

Body Function	Normal Microbiome Functions	Consequences of Compromised Function
Control of microorganisms	Prevent pathogenic infection through microbiome inertia.	Tendency toward food infections, bowel disorders, SIBO, ulcers.
Gut lining health	Produce an energy source for gut epithelium.	Unhealthy gut epithelium, malabsorption, hypovitaminosis, leaky gut, ulcers, anemia, food intolerance, some allergies.
Gut motility	Stimulate normal gut motility.	Lazy gut, constipation, diarrhea.
Nutrient status	Synthesize certain required nutrients— essential amino acids, some vitamins (K, B_{12}).	Lack of some nutrients, anemia, bleeding tendency, unhealthy gut epithelium.
Immune system	Maintain a healthy immune system.	Immune disorders— allergies, autoimmune diseases, higher probability of some cancers.

Note: Research continues to uncover additional microbiota functions and their associations with diseases beyond those listed above.

Appendix 1: Table 3.2. Normal microbiome functions and consequences of compromised function

Your immune cells are constantly interacting with your resident bacteria, to the point where it can be said that the microbiome defines them. Considering an impressive 70% of all immune cells are in the gut, this explains the microbiome's central role in our strategy to combat autoimmune diseases and allergies. You cannot have a robust immune system without a healthy microbiome.

See also:

• Appendix 1 ➤ Table 3.2

MAINTAINING A RESILIENT MICROBIOME

Factors That Keep Your Microbiome Healthy

Factors:	We Cover These In:
Digestive Process, Stomach Acid, Bile, Saliva, Mastication	Key 1. Dysbiosis: Repopulate the Microbiome.
Food Ingredients and Eating Habits	Key 1. Dysbiosis: Repopulate the Microbiome.
Bacterial Ecosystem Inertia and Resilience	Key 1. Dysbiosis: Repopulate the Microbiome.
Intestinal Immune System Status	Key 2. Inflammation: Reduce.
Digestive System Epithelium	Key 3. Leaky Gut: Repair.
Gastrointestinal Motility	Key 4. Lazy Gut: Reawaken.
Continuous Contact with Germs	Key 5. Factors Beyond Digestive Health: Recondition. ➤ The Hygiene Paradox: When Cleaning Backfires.
Climate and Microclimate	Key 5. Factors Beyond Digestive Health: Recondition. ➤ Environment and Climate: Where You Live Matters.

Appendix 1: Table 3.3. Factors that keep your microbiome healthy

Just as other body parts adjust to changes—your skin darkens under the sun, and muscles strengthen through exercise—the microbiome evolves in response to shifts in your body and surroundings. Everything from your diet, state of health, travel experiences, or a new workplace can alter its composition. In a healthy person, these changes are typically well-managed and balanced. However, sometimes, these adaptations can be derailed and cause damage instead.

When such imbalances occur, the immune system often bears the brunt of the impact, leading to autoimmune diseases, allergies, and certain types of cancers. This interaction between the microbiome and the immune system affects the entire body. Thus, healing requires more than a one-dimensional strategy. Refer to Table 3.3 for a detailed list of the factors we will explore for restoring your gut microbiome.

Each component plays an integral role in creating the microbiome ecosystem. We will discuss these factors in detail in later sections of the book. For now, let us focus on the direct impact of food and digestion on the microbiome.

HEALING AN ECOSYSTEM

How do you heal a whole ecosystem? The answer lies in the unique approach of the *5R+ System*. Unlike most methods that rely solely on food and probiotics, this approach recognizes that merely tweaking bacteria levels is not enough.

 To truly transform your microbiome, you need to rebuild its entire ecosystem.

This program will walk you through effective strategies for achieving this. Dealing with autoimmune diseases is complex. It requires self-discipline and time. Some might notice improvements in just a few months. For others, particularly those who have been battling with an autoimmune condition for longer—usually older adults—it may take up to 3-4 years. It is a long journey, but like everyone else on this road, you'll start seeing positive changes along the way, no matter how long it takes. Breaking may be faster than fixing, but fixing is within your grasp.

Every effort to change encounters resistance—*inertia* is always at play. This is true for the microbiome as well. This section explores how inertia can be both a hurdle and a helper in your journey.

See also:
- Appendix 1 ➤ Figure 3.3.1

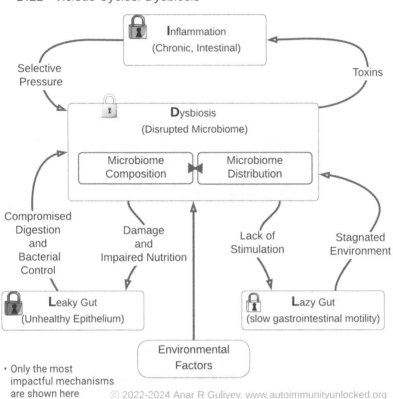

DILL+ Vicious Cycles: Dysbiosis

Appendix 1: Figure 3.3.1. DILL+ Vicious Cycles: Dysbiosis

OVERCOMING MICROBIOTA INERTIA: CONQUEST OR IMMIGRATION

The microbiome is a fickle beast, and its effects vary significantly from person to person. For instance, two people eat the same meal and drink the same water. One feels great afterward, but the other ends up with a digestive infection.

Let's add more detail: this meal had seen better days and brought along some microscopic troublemakers. A healthy microbiome can handle such occasional dietary assaults. Like any well-balanced ecosystem, the microbiota possesses *inertia*—it is resilient and tends to remain unchanged.

> **A healthy, well-established microbiome community doesn't easily succumb to random harmful factors.**

In other words, an occasional unhealthy choice is unlikely to cause significant damage. Yet, continuous and repeated attacks can gradually erode this microbiome fortress, allowing harmful elements to establish themselves in their new home—your ecosystem.

> The inertia of an ecosystem refers to its capacity to withstand changes when faced with disruptions or stress. This concept is akin to resilience, which is about the system's ability to recover and revert to its original state. While experts differentiate between inertia and resilience, for the sake of simplicity in our discussion, we'll use the term 'inertia' to encompass the overall stability and reaction of the microbiome.

The microbiota is resilient, meaning it can recover from minor disturbances. To significantly alter the ecosystem's composition, the disrupting force must be strong enough to break through its defenses or be a consistent, slow erosion over a long time. Picture a city inhabited by defensive residents, ready to destroy random intruders and resist intermittent assaults. The only way to change this population is either through a rapid, massive invasion or a continuous influx of immigrants over many years. This analogy mirrors the situation with pathogenic bacteria: they stand little chance of survival if they arrive in small numbers or only occasionally—the established microbiome can hold them off. However, a significant infection or a long-term unhealthy lifestyle can weaken the microbiome, making it vulnerable to intruders. Examples of these two scenarios in the microbiota can be:

- **Conquest:** acute infection, food poisoning, and trauma.
- **Immigration:** unhealthy diet, bad lifestyle habits, chronic poisoning, and long-term exposure to pathogens.

This principle is not exclusive to microbiomes; it is seen in other ecosystems, too. For example, a forest can withstand occasional hunting or brief droughts. Nature is resilient and can bounce back, provided the damage is not too extreme or prolonged.

Your microbiome's defense system is complex. As the initial layer of protection is breached, you will likely experience digestive issues. If the damage persists, these problems can escalate, leading to immune complications like allergies and more serious autoimmune disorders. The ecosystem's inertia attempts to counter these advances to the best of its ability. A diverse and robust microbiome—like a dense, varied forest rather than a single-crop farm—offers stronger resistance against harmful changes. It neutralizes random intruders and manages problematic food, often without you even noticing, though sometimes you might feel slight discomfort or have a brief bout of diarrhea. Hunter-gatherers are a perfect example of this. Their varied and robust microbiomes allow them to consume spoiled meat and impure water without harm, a stark contrast to those living in a more modern setting who might struggle even with safe foods.

Thus, inertia is a positive factor in a **healthy microbiome**, as it helps maintain stability and prevents harmful deviations. However, for people with *dysbiosis* (imbalance in gut bacteria), this inertia works against them. It preserves an ecosystem of sickness populated by harmful microbes, hindering the return to good health.

Indeed, many hover between health and illness, where the ecosystem's condition is not so bad as to manifest as disease, but not strong and stable either. Imagine it is balancing on the edge of a cliff—a minor exposure to pathogens can disrupt this fragile equilibrium. In an unhealthy, weak microbiome, even a tiny disturbance—like contaminated food or an episode of inflammation or epithelial damage—can cause significant issues. Harmful bacteria and fungi can take over this vulnerable niche, establishing a new, opposite inertia. This shift will actively work against the body, preventing the good bacteria from easily colonizing the flipped ecosystem.

The key is cultivating a healthy, varied microbiome with the right combination of diverse bacteria, akin to a self-sustaining forest. Such a microbiome is well-equipped to manage infections or the occasional indulgence in unhealthy food. To help repopulate your microbiome, I recommend naturally fermented foods rather than probiotic supplements. The reason is that supplements contain fewer viable bacteria due to extended shelf lives, potentially diminishing their impact on your microbial balance. Additionally, industrialized manufacturing processes result in a low variety of bacterial strains, further limiting their ability to support a diverse gut microbiome. Conversely, fermented foods teem with active, beneficial microbes that are more likely to endure and effect tangible changes in your system. Because DIY fermentation inevitably occurs under different conditions each time, it brings natural variety, which is essential for your gut. Check out our *Bonus* section for some delicious recipes. Incorporating these foods into your diet, along with our other strategic keys, can lead to rapid and noticeable health improvements as you navigate towards unlocking your "autoimmune shackles."

Our approach reshapes your microbiome from an unstable or unhealthy state to a stable and healthy condition. The bacterial population's resistance to the change is similar to pushing a wheelbarrow over a hill; it is hard at first, but once you're over the top, inertia works in your favor. That's why I recommend the strictest diet during your initial active healing period.

I've said it before, and I'm saying it again: the process will require time and patience, but the results are worth it. A restored and healthy ecosystem within your body offers immense benefits in the long run. While I don't recommend returning to junk food, you'll find that you can gradually reintroduce healthy foods that previously triggered adverse reactions. However, take it slow. In my case, after my rheumatoid arthritis had been in remission for a few years, I tried adding nuts back into my diet. It turned out this was premature and led to a flare-up. Only after a few more years could I enjoy them again without any problems.

See also:

• Key 1 ➢ Probiotics

• Bonus 2. The Art of Fermentation: Delicious Vegetable and Dairy Probiotics Recipes.

AFTERMATH OF MICROBIAL INVASIONS

As mentioned, a massive invasion can quickly overcome the body's natural inertia. In food poisoning, for example, a severe intestinal infection disrupts your microbiome and damages the gut epithelium. The toxins released can harm the nerve cells in your intestines, negatively impacting motility. This domino effect can break down several defense mechanisms, creating multiple DILL+ locks and potentially leading to dysbiosis and autoimmune diseases. For example, infections like *brucellosis* and *shigellosis* often trigger arthritis. Then there is the issue of antibiotics. While they are used to fight harmful infections, they can also inadvertently threaten your immune system by destroying many of your beneficial bacteria.

We often see patients develop conditions like rheumatoid arthritis, lupus, or ulcerative colitis after an acute illness that disrupted their microbial ecosystem. But don't worry; even after such a severe infection, you can still turn things around. The human gut is remarkably resilient and capable of regenerating its cells, including nerve cells—this stands in stark contrast to the brain's neurons, which possess limited regenerative capacity.

Once an acute infection is treated, particularly in cases involving antibiotics, our 5R+ approach can successfully restore the immune system and the balance in the gut microbiome. Start this restoration process soon after recovering from the illness, as delaying it could lead to more damage.

These blitzkrieg invasions are a problem. Yet, dysbiosis more often develops subtly through "immigration"—a gradual inflow of newcomers that shifts the population over time. The good news? The restoration strategies are similar in both scenarios, and our system is designed to address each situation effectively.

THE TWO DIMENSIONS OF MICROBIOME HEALTH

There are two main microbiome dimensions that we must rebuild and maintain:

- **Microbiome Composition:** The variety of microorganisms in your gut. Which types are present, and in what proportions? It's a diverse crowd—some bacteria are beneficial, others are harmful, and many fall somewhere in between.
- **Microbiome Distribution:** The location of the microorganisms within your digestive system and how densely they are distributed. For example, the colon should be packed with trillions of bacteria, whereas the stomach and upper small intestine have very few.

Microbiome composition and distribution are closely linked—if one is disrupted, the other is also likely to be affected. Fortunately, we have strategies that effectively target both these dimensions.

DIMENSION 1: MICROBIOME COMPOSITION

WHO LIVES INSIDE US

The microbiome's composition refers to the type and number of different bacterial species it contains. Your gut alone is home to over a thousand varieties. This organ is unique to each individual, varying more than any other organ—even between identical twins. Your microbiome today is different from what it was last year. When discussing "diseases of modernity," like those affecting the immune system, it is interesting to note that the microbiome is the only part of the human body that has undergone significant changes in recent decades. Numerous factors influence these shifts—your lifestyle, diet, health status, home environment, and even your job.

As already mentioned, genetics plays a role in predisposing people to autoimmune diseases. Still, while you can't alter your DNA, the genetic makeup of your microbiome, given its malleability, is another story. It is constantly changing. Moving from India to the US (where mac-and-cheese replaces biryani on your table), switching from urban to rural living, changing careers, or even getting a new pet can significantly impact your microbiome, for better or worse. I've seen people develop autoimmune diseases after moving from the Mediterranean to the US or Canada. And while diet is a key influencing factor, it is just one of many we will explore throughout this book.

Thankfully, you don't need to meticulously analyze the composition of your microbiota and attempt to balance thousands of bacterial species. That would be an overwhelming task! Instead, we'll focus on a principle backed by numerous studies as the most effective strategy—**Diversity**.

 The goal is a varied and diverse microbiome.

CAMELS IN THE JUNGLE – WHY PROBIOTICS ARE NOT ENOUGH

The habitat you create in your gut determines which bacteria flourish, becoming integral to the complex ecosystem that influences your cells and overall organism.

Consider this analogy: if you moved Arabian camels to the Amazon jungle, they wouldn't survive because it is not their natural habitat. The climate, vegetation, and even the local wildlife are entirely different from what they need to thrive, not to mention the diseases they might face. You would need to drastically alter the environment to make it possible for camels to live in the jungle. Similarly, adding more bacteria to your gut with probiotics doesn't automatically change its bacterial composition. Even radical repopulation approaches like *fecal microbial transplants* often don't have lasting effects. Many patients undergo this unpleasant procedure repeatedly without adopting the necessary lifestyle adjustments.

Lasting improvement will only occur when you transform the entire ecosystem over time. Think again about the differences between the desert and the rainforest. It's not just the plants the camels eat but also factors like humidity, wind, water, and soil that matter. In the same way, your gut ecosystem needs more than just health-promoting food. The microbiome and its ecosystem are central to the DILL+ system. That's why our 5R+ strategies address a wide range of "levers," from gut motility to the health of your epithelial cells and even your hormones—all crucial for achieving solid and enduring results.

See also:
- Key 1 ➤ Actively Repopulate ➤ Probiotics

VARIETY — FARMLAND VS. FOREST

Consider the differences between a wild, diverse forest and a uniform farmland blanketed with endless rows of corn. The forest exhibits a natural *resilience* thanks to its richly varied ecosystem. In contrast, farmers must constantly work hard to maintain their 'monoculture' fields. This cornfield is like a one-legged stool—a little nudge, and it topples over. One harsh season, be it drought, pests, or a severe storm, could be the end of the cornfield. Ultimately, if left undisturbed by human intervention, nature will reclaim the land, naturally transforming it back into a diverse and varied ecosystem. Sadly, many modern individuals resemble the cornfield more than the forest, with their microbiomes needing more variety. This similarity is why many people experience issues like stomach upset from common foods and, in some cases, more severe digestive and immune problems.

It is even more evident when we look at the differences in diversity among various cultures. Fascinating research highlights the stark contrast in microbiome diversity between individuals in modern Western societies and those living in more traditional cultures. Studies reveal that hunter-gatherer communities, such as the Hadza in Africa and certain groups in South America, boast a much more versatile array of gut bacteria compared to people in countries like Italy. The studies also showed that the typical American microbiome is even less diverse, a problem closely linked to our modern lifestyle. See Figures 3.4 and 3.5.

There are many reasons why people in traditional societies, who still adhere to age-old practices, have a far richer microbiome diversity than those in more modern cultures. They eat only fresh produce and unprocessed foods and spend a lot of time outdoors. Whether engaging in agricultural work or walking through forests, these people naturally encounter a variety of germs, which help strengthen their immune systems and enhance microbiome diversity. Historically, allergies and autoimmune diseases were almost non-existent. However, with modern lifestyle changes, there has been a marked increase in these conditions, with some countries reporting prevalence rates exceeding 20% of their population.

Just as a monoculture farm is vulnerable, so is a microbiome that lacks variety. Our goal is to enhance the diversity within the microbiome, fostering an environment that supports a number of beneficial bacterial species that, regrettably, have become nearly extinct in modern people.

A weakened microbiome becomes an easy target for harmful pathogens and creates an imbalanced environment for immune cells. Digestive disorders like gluten sensitivity, food intolerances, and irregular bowel movements have become so common that they are often considered normal. It's striking to see how frequently people in the U.S. suffer from stomach cramps after eating something as simple as cabbage.

 Common does not mean normal!

A diverse microbiome introduces a level of forgiveness to your dietary choices. A varied and resilient microbiome with strong inertia can tolerate occasional "bad" food choices. You might currently react to a small piece of gluten-containing bread or a glass of milk. After repopulating your microbiome, though, even the odd junk food won't cause lasting damage—your good microbes will act as a protective shield. Of course, I don't recommend returning to a poor diet, as this will lead you back to the vicious circle of an unhealthy ecosystem.

 A healthy microbiome is like a diverse forest, not a monoculture farm.

Having established this theoretical groundwork, let's move on to practical strategies for nurturing a healthy *Microbiota Composition*. In the next chapter, we'll focus on actively repopulating the microbiome before turning our attention to the second dimension, *Microbiome Distribution*.

See also:

• Appendix 1 ➢ Figures 3.4, 3.5

ACTIVELY REPOPULATE

Think about your lawn for a moment. Grass needs water, sunlight, and fertilization to grow, but weeds thrive on the same elements. Regular mowing helps control weeds. However, more action is required to tackle these unwelcome intruders effectively. Creating a robust foundation with the appropriate type of grass is vital. The dense green carpet will be a natural barrier against weed invasion in your yard. In nature, empty spaces are like open invitations for new inhabitants. Any bare spots in your lawn can quickly turn into hotspots for weeds. However, a lush, dense lawn occupies all *ecological niches*, leaving little opportunity for unwanted plants to move in.

Your gut's ecosystem is similar to a garden: a lush, dense population of beneficial bacteria ensures all ecological niches are filled and in balance. Just as regular mowing, the right weed killers and carefully chosen fertilizers help grass outcompete weeds, maintaining good gut motility, proper digestive juices, and foods providing nutrients for the good microorganisms support a healthy microbiome. At the same time, foods that feed harmful bacteria must be avoided or at least minimized.

These elements help rebuild a normal microbiome, a cornerstone of a healthy immune system. Diversity ensures that a wide range of beneficial bacteria occupy multiple ecosystem niches in the gut, leaving no room for unwanted germs. Scientists are still exploring the intricacies of this process, but one thing is clear: an unvaried microbiome is fragile. It leads to immune system imbalances and is easily disturbed by dietary shifts or pathogenic bacteria.

 A low-diversity ecosystem is fragile and easily disrupted.

BUILDING A HEALTHY COMMUNITY

The factors facilitating the *Repopulation of the Microbiome* include:

- Probiotics—food *with* beneficial bacteria.
- Prebiotics—food *for* beneficial bacteria.
- Wide variety of specific raw, whole food ingredients.
- Simultaneous correction of other DILL+ factors by applying all 5R+ keys.

PROBIOTICS

Probiotic supplements have become very popular in recent years. This surge is driven by the growing fascination with the topic of the gut microbiome, turning probiotics into a multibillion-dollar industry.

While they have their uses, they are often less effective than advertised. Increasing research suggests that simply popping a daily pill is not enough to tackle the issue and is far from being a natural approach. Several obstacles stand in the way of probiotics successfully colonizing the gut, with *inertia* being the greatest challenge. Supplements frequently include dormant or weakened strains. They might not be robust enough to impact the existing ecosystem, an unavoidable trade-off for their longer shelf life. Also, the stomach produces acid, and the liver produces bile as a defense against foreign invaders. To survive this "double firewall," some probiotic supplements are contained in stomach acid-resistant capsules. However, for these supplements to be effective, large numbers of active, viable bacteria must be delivered to the gut daily, mixed with a large volume of food. Even more alarming is that standardized manufacturing processes create a limited variety of bacterial strains. Research suggests these industrialized supple-ments may even reduce microbiome diversity. While prescription probiotics offer benefits in certain instances, such limitations can restrict their effectiveness.

There's a better method as ancient as the history of food itself: Many traditional cuisines feature probiotic-rich fermented products boasting a wide variety of bacterial strains. Homemade and artisanal fermented foods are naturally made under varied fermentation condi-tions. They also allow you to improvise with different combinations of vegetables and herbs, resulting in an even broader array of bacterial strains—much more than any manufacturer could offer. Just as hand-made crafts are always different, the microbial population in your jars will never be the same, unlike factory-produced items. Even high-quality industrially fermented products made using standardized processes with uniform strains tend to have less variety. Surprisingly, many commercial brands of pickles contain no living bacteria at all.

 Industrially made probiotics vs. naturally fermented vegetables is like comparing a wheelchair to a race car.

Studies consistently show that fresh, traditionally prepared probi-otic foods offer superior diversity and viability than their manufac-tured counterparts. The *Bonus* section provides easy-to-follow recipes for creating these at home. Regularly incorporating homemade fermented foods into your diet can gradually shift your microbiome composition, overcoming its inertia. There's no strict portion or schedule—it is not a drug, just food that aids healing. Go with what feels right: a couple of tablespoons or a cup. In the initial phase of active healing, I advise higher daily doses, which you can reduce later based on your preference.

See also:

• Bonus 2. The Art of Fermentation: Delicious Vegetable and Dairy Probiotics Recipes.

FERMENTED VEGETABLES AND PICKLES

Naturally fermented foods are cornerstones in many traditional diets: from *sauerkraut* in Germany to *turshu* in Turkey, and Korean *kimchi*, to Japanese *natto*. Each culture has its own take on these fermented treasures. Beyond enhancing the microbiome, these flavorful dishes are powerful antifungal agents, crucial in tackling mold growth issues often found in severe autoimmune conditions. Mold leads to a particularly unpleasant type of dysbiosis, which can be challenging but not impossible to overcome, a topic we will cover later.

Not all fermented products are equal. The potency of pickled vegetables varies. For instance, some spicy pickles preserved in oil and hot pepper, common in Indian cuisine, were initially designed to endure hot and humid conditions. While they undergo some fermentation, they are often less effective for our intended purposes.

Also, traditionally made pickles are an excellent source of good bacteria. Yet, most supermarket pickles don't offer any probiotic benefits. They are not genuinely fermented; instead, they are simply soaked in salt and vinegar. While not necessarily unhealthy—unless loaded with additives like sugar, artificial flavors, colors, or taste enhancers—they don't qualify as probiotic foods.

The gut health benefits of naturally fermented foods are undeniable. Learn how to make your own, using the recipes from *Bonus 2*. Experiment with them: feel free to improvise with different vegetable and herb combinations to enjoy a wider variety of probiotics, literally infusing new life into your meals. While you don't need to have these foods every day, aim for several servings weekly. Use a variety of herbs and fermented vegetables to flavor your meals instead of store-bought dressings packed with long lists of synthetic ingredients that challenge your knowledge of chemistry. Homemade or authentically fermented products are far superior to shelf-stable, store-bought versions.

Warning: If you are dealing with hypertension or kidney issues or your doctor has advised you to limit your sodium or salt intake, choose low-salt recipes and be mindful of portion sizes. Refrain from adding extra salt to your food. Always consult your doctor for personalized advice.

See also:

• Key 1 ➤ Fungi: Mold and Yeast

. . .

FERMENTED DAIRY

Many with autoimmune issues often need to steer clear of dairy initially. However, as you progress in your healing, you might be able to reintroduce it slowly. Here are a few considerations:

- Cow milk often increases inflammation.
- Sensitivities to fresh milk are more common than reactions to fermented dairy products.
- Cows are treated with hormones and antibiotics more often and in higher doses than sheep or goats.
- Goat or sheep milk products are a better choice because they are less likely to trigger food intolerances or adverse reactions.
- Always opt for products from animals never treated with hormones and antibiotics.

A healthy microbiome can typically process dairy well, especially when all DILL+ components are enhanced. Still, it is essential to proceed with caution during the *Reintroduction* stage. Start with a small amount and monitor your body's response for any adverse reactions over the next 4-5 days. If you choose to avoid dairy entirely, that's okay, too. Consuming fermented vegetables is a great way to restore gut health for those who prefer or need to avoid dairy permanently.

A wide variety of fermented dairy products is available. Unfortunately, not all offer probiotic benefits or qualify as healthy food. First, be wary of those flashy products from the modern food industry that crowd supermarket shelves, promising intense flavors through artificial ingredients or added sugars. The manufacture of these products is anything but natural, often relying on starches and additives to achieve the perfect texture and preservatives for a longer shelf life. My rule of thumb is simple:

 I don't eat or drink anything that didn't exist a thousand years ago.

Most importantly, steer clear of foods devised during the modern marketing era, where the race to outdo competitors with attractive pricing and appeal has become a sophisticated, dominating force. Avoid sweetened dairy products—the combination of milk and sugar is a favorite of many harmful bacteria. Instead, choose whole, natural foods free from additives, with minimal ingredient lists. They might taste a bit bland compared to processed foods, but you can always enhance them with herbs or berries—fresh, dried, or frozen. Remember, no preservatives means a shorter shelf life, which is crucial for the products' probiotic properties.

 Be the commander of your taste preferences.

In English, 'yogurt' is the common term for most fermented dairy products, but many varieties exist. Since ancient times, traditional pastoral cultures have created a wide range of artisanal dairy foods integral to their diets. Try *qatiq* and *laban*, similar to plain Greek, Turkish, or Bulgarian yogurt; *ayran*, a thinner, drinkable version; or *labneh*, a thick, creamy strained yogurt cheese. When buying these, choose ones without starch or other additives. Better yet, try making them yourself —it's easier than you think.

See also:

• Key 1 ➤ Chemical Additives and Toxins in Our Food

CHEESE

Not every cheese is a good source of probiotics, nor are they all beneficial for health. Unfortunately, this includes many popular varieties. Steer clear of:

- **Processed cheeses**, including the creamy, spreadable types and those commonly used in pizzas. Processed foods often lose nutritional value and contain unnatural additives.
- **Non-dairy cheese**, gaining popularity among vegans and those with lactose intolerance, is also processed, often soy-based, and carries its own concerns.

- **Cheese with fungus**—whether due to spoilage or as a feature in mold-ripened varieties such as blue cheese, camembert, and brie. These fungi can significantly harm the microbiome. Intestinal fungal overgrowth is a particularly challenging issue to address.

Probiotic-rich cheeses are typically those that haven't been heat-treated or industrially processed and are free from additives and preservatives. Aged cheeses like cheddar, gouda, edam, and kashkaval can retain viable bacteria, which diminish over time. Fresh cheeses— such as mozzarella, feta, bryndza, labneh, chèvre, paneer, caciocavallo, halloumi, artisanal sheep and goat cheeses, and some cottage cheeses —are a better source of beneficial bacteria. They are often preserved in brine, a much better method than chemical additives. However, these cheeses have a limited shelf life, just like any other probiotic-rich food. And, if you're dealing with even a slight dairy sensitivity—which is likely if you have a *Leaky Gut*—cheese, due to its high protein content, might worsen inflammation. It is wise to hold off on cheese until you are past the active healing phase. After that, you can carefully start reintroducing it into your diet in small amounts.

See also:
- Key 1 ➣ Chemical Additives and Toxins in Our Food
- Key 5 ➣ Xenoestrogens
- Key 1 ➣ Fungi: Mold and Yeast

FERMENTED FOOD RECIPES

It is worth emphasizing: for probiotic-rich foods, the fresher and more traditionally prepared, the better. These "old-style" methods cultivate richer strains of bacteria than uniform, industrial processes. To spark some DIY enthusiasm, you have complimentary access to my collection of recipes. Check out the *Bonus 2* section, *The Art of Fermentation: Delicious Vegetable and Dairy Probiotics Recipes*, included with this book.

With some practice, you'll quickly get the hang of making these at home. Once you're comfortable, you can have some fun and experiment with your creations. You are doing more than just enhancing taste; every tweak—different vegetables, herbs, spices, or ingredient ratios—creates a distinct bacterial profile. Each unique blend you concoct contributes to a more robust and more diverse microbiome.

Fecal Microbial Transplantation: Success or Temporary Fix?

Probiotics hold the key to better health. There's a medical procedure that distinctly demonstrates their potential: *fecal microbiota transplantation (FMT)*. It involves transferring bacteria from a healthy individual's colon to someone with poor gut health. FMT has recently emerged as a powerful tool to mitigate many autoimmune conditions. Numerous cases have shown outstanding outcomes, illustrating the benefits of enriching the microbiome with beneficial bacteria.

Our first 5R+ key, *Repopulate*, has a similar goal through a more natural and consistent method. This approach transforms the entire ecosystem, creating an environment where the beneficial bacteria can thrive and successfully compete. If not consistently supported, the microbiome and your overall health could revert to their prior ailing state. This is a common scenario among FMT patients who don't change their lifestyle; they often find themselves needing repeated treatments. The next chapter will explore ways to nourish and empower the "good" bacteria for optimal performance.

FEEDING YOUR ALLIES

Incorporating probiotic bacteria into your diet is the first step towards a robust microbiome. The next is to sustain their positive effect on your gut and overall health by feeding them properly. There is a catch, though. The foods that support probiotics should not simultaneously encourage the growth of pathogenic bacteria. That's why a carefully chosen mix of *prebiotics*—the food that bacteria feed on—and other selected nutrients is essential, which is covered in this chapter.

Prebiotics

By definition, prebiotics are food for bacteria, fueling their growth and activity. While almost any carbohydrate can serve this purpose, not all are equally beneficial. Foods rich in readily fermentable sugars or starches, especially those low in fiber, may negatively impact your microbiome. One possible consequence is the excessive growth of bacteria in the upper small intestine, leading to conditions like *Small Intestinal Bacterial Overgrowth (SIBO)* or *Lazy Gut*. Frequently, SIBO leads to negative responses to prebiotic vegetables, such as stomach upset, gas, bloating, and cramps. Though sometimes it can stay hidden, and immune issues are the only signs. If you have SIBO or Lazy gut—which often go hand in hand—moderate your prebiotic intake until you notice significant progress in resolving these conditions. I'll discuss the arsenal you can use against these common yet often undetected issues later.

Good prebiotic foods should possess two essential qualities:

- They must be high in fiber to promote quicker digestive transit.
- They must be rich in specific bioactive compounds and enzymes that regulate bacterial growth rate.

Fruits, legumes, and raw vegetables are the best sources of prebiotics for your bacteria. Herbs and bitter vegetables stand out for their exceptional effectiveness. Instead of reaching for cookies or cake, try mint, arugula, or radishes. Acquire a taste for bitter veggies and make your food choices work in your favor.

 Love the food that loves you back.

See also:
- Key 1 ➤ Healthy Digestion to Fix Microbiota Distribution
- Key 4 ➤ Your Food and Gut Motility

GOOD BITTER TRUTH

Often neglected in our diets, bitter vegetables play a crucial role in gut health. The compounds that give some herbs and vegetables their bitter flavor are also natural bacterial inhibitors, slowing down their growth. This is why bitter veggies generally spoil more slowly than their non-bitter counterparts. In the gut, these inhibitors effectively curb the rapid multiplication of aggressive bacterial strains, allowing other species the chance to settle in and thrive.

Imagine a loaded pickup truck and a fast sports car in a speed contest. On a smooth highway, the pickup truck stands no chance. Yet, on a rough, pothole-ridden backroad, where speed is limited for both, it competes more effectively. Similarly, some bacteria multiply faster than others. Adding "obstacles to the race" caps the speed, giving a greater variety of strains a chance to hold and thrive. A diet rich in raw vegetables, herbs, and spices is high in antimicrobial compounds that can level the playing field in your gut just as the potholed road does for the vehicles, creating a more diverse microbial community. This fundamental concept and the importance of including foods that help regulate bacterial growth for a more varied and balanced gut microbiome will be revisited and emphasized later.

 Diverse, healthy microbiota thrive in a gut akin to a rugged backcountry, not a lawn of sweets and starch.

Bitter vegetables have been valued as potent digestive allies since ancient times. Interestingly, bitter taste receptors are located not only in your mouth but also in your intestines and colon. Thankfully, we don't taste food in our colons! These receptors do much more than sense flavors; they regulate various digestive processes and moderate appetite, aiding in weight management. The large intestine, the organ with the most dense colonization of bacteria, also has the highest concentration of these receptors. This hints at the importance of bitter vegetables in maintaining a healthy gut microbiome and promoting overall digestive health.

Raw vegetables, including bitter ones, served with herbs in a mixed salad, are a delicious way to enhance your health. Additionally, always pair meat or fish meals with fresh bitter veggies to aid digestion.

Here are some recommended ingredients from our *Blue and Green Food Baskets*:

- Radishes: all varieties, including daikon and turnips.
- Onion family: onions, leeks, garlic, scallions, chives.
- Ginger.
- Leafy greens: arugula, watercress, endive, kale, lettuce, Swiss chard, collard, mustard, and turnip greens.
- Cabbage family: cabbage, cauliflower, broccoli, Brussels sprouts, kohlrabi, bok choy.

As we'll see below, it is best to eat vegetables raw.

 Always combine meat or fish with a generous amount of raw, bitter vegetables and herbs.

See also:
- Key 1 ➤ Stomach Acid
- Key 1 ➤ Bile and Liver Health
- Appendix 1 ➤ Table 4.4
- Bonus 3. Food Baskets: Foods Ranked by Their Impact on the Gut-Microbiome-Immune Ecosystem

DEAD OR ALIVE — ENZYMES IN YOUR FOOD

Fruits and vegetables are rich in enzymes and bioactive compounds with many functions, including regulating microorganism growth. In the wild, these compounds prevent plants from rotting while alive. Even after being harvested, the enzymes in vegetables remain active for some time. The enduring vitality of plants, even post-harvest, is quite remarkable, especially when compared to animals—consider, for instance, how a bouquet of cut flowers can survive in a vase for many days. However, cooking at high temperatures breaks down these complex components, leaving vegetables truly "dead." That's why cooked veggies spoil more quickly than raw ones and can encourage rapid bacterial growth in the small intestine.

> Enzymes are proteins that function as catalysts
> in living organisms, speeding up vital chemical
> reactions such as digestion, metabolism,
> defense, growth, and many more.

On the other hand, raw vegetables retain their natural defenses, enabling a gradual digestion and nutrient absorption process throughout the small intestine. Some nutrients will travel all the way to the colon, the microbiome's primary residence, feeding the bacteria there.

The benefits of eating raw vegetables have been recognized for centuries. It was once thought that enzymes in uncooked produce aided digestion, but now we understand that they regulate the microbiome. Beyond enzymes, plants have other heat-sensitive potent antimicrobial compounds that target specific bacteria. For example, herbs, seeds, and spices are often rich in essential oils, which, like enzymes, can be destroyed by cooking.

 Most of our food should consist of raw plants, and most plants can be eaten raw.

In contrast, mechanical preparation methods like cutting, mixing, freezing, and drying generally preserve the beneficial chemistry of plants. So, how you prepare your food impacts your digestive process and microbiome. Whenever possible, use non-thermal methods for most of your food preparation.

While more research is needed to fully grasp how eating raw vegetables impacts the microbiome, current findings are promising, suggesting increased diversity and better distribution of gut bacteria. One recent study on healthy individuals revealed noticeable differences in just three days.

Digesting Raw Vegetables

A healthy digestive system typically handles raw vegetables with ease. However, if your gut and microbiome are compromised, you might face some difficulties initially. Don't worry—with consistent application of the 5R+ strategies, these issues should slowly diminish as your gut lining repairs itself.

You can take various steps to ease the load on your stomach and intestines while retaining the essential nutrients often sacrificed in heat-based cooking. The first is to choose foods that nourish a healthy microbiome while being mechanically gentle on your sensitive gut. Start with soft and juicy vegetables like spinach, parsley, fennel, squash, and cucumbers to ease digestion. Fruits and bitter vegetables, such as arugula, kale, mustard greens, and onions, are also excellent choices—use the options from our *Green Basket*. Shredding or cutting these foods into tiny pieces can further aid digestion, reducing mechanical irritation. And remember, there's no getting around good old chewing. After all, your stomach hasn't grown any teeth!

For those with conditions like *IBS (Irritable Bowel Syndrome)*, *Crohn's*, *ulcerative colitis*, or *IBD (Inflammatory Bowel Disease)*, digesting raw vegetables can pose an even greater challenge due to the already damaged epithelium. Consider blending your veggies into smoothies in these cases for easier digestion. Blending won't change their chemistry, but it will make them gentler on your gut while offering all the benefits of raw food. Add herbs, spices, or fermented pickles and their juice to improve the taste. It will also supercharge your smoothie with antifungal and probiotic properties. Small amounts of turmeric and ginger can also aid in reducing inflammation. These ingredients have shown benefits for conditions like Crohn's disease, but always consult your doctor first.

As you consistently follow the 5R+ approach, your gut health and microbiome will gradually improve, allowing you to enjoy a wider variety of raw vegetables. Apart from a few exceptions (like potatoes), most vegetables can and should be eaten raw.

 Ideally, more than half of your diet should consist of raw vegetables, fruits, nuts, and seeds.

See also:
• Key 3 ➢ Quasi-Elemental Diet

- Key 2 ➤ Spices and Herbs to Reduce Inflammation
- Bonus 3. Food Baskets: Foods Ranked by Their Impact on the Gut-Microbiome-Immune Ecosystem

FROZEN, DRIED, SALTED — PRESERVING RAW PRODUCE

Freezing is the best method for preserving food, mainly because it keeps most enzymes and bioactive compounds intact. The only downside to freezing is mechanical damage—ice crystals can rupture cell walls, altering the texture and taste of thawed vegetables. However, this isn't always a problem. Berries, for example, are just as delicious frozen as fresh—super convenient and always a tasty treat. Just remember, foods spoil more quickly once thawed, so eating them soon after is best.

Interestingly, frozen foods can sometimes be more nutritious than fresh ones. "Fresh" vegetables often undergo a lengthy journey from farm to market, sometimes spanning up to two weeks. This usually means they're picked before fully ripening, leading them to do so en route in a truck instead of naturally on the plant under the sunshine. That's why I recommend frozen berries—picked at peak ripeness and frozen quickly to preserve their nutrients. This is also why local produce trumps imported goods—it travels less, preserving more nutrients.

Next up is drying—almost as good as freezing, particularly for fruits. Salt is sometimes used to speed up the drying process, slightly altering the chemical composition of foods. Always rinse off any excess salt, especially if you have high blood pressure or kidney issues. Traditional preservation methods like these mostly maintain the food's nutritional value, unlike modern methods that often involve the addition of harmful chemicals. Removing those residues is trickier than simply washing away a bit of salt.

Ozone preservation is another noteworthy technique. It uses atomic oxygen to kill bacteria, avoiding harmful chemical residues. This method ensures food stays safe and fresh for an extended period. Ozone devices are now available for domestic use and offer a convenient solution to extend food's shelf life in your kitchen.

. . .

POLYPHENOLS: THE COLORFUL PATH TO A DIVERSE MICROBIOME

Have you ever thought about why your plate should look like a rainbow? Beyond the visual appeal, colorful foods are rich in polyphenols, offering potent health benefits. The vibrant colors in many fruits and vegetables come from these nutritious chemicals.

> Polyphenols, found abundantly in plant-based foods, are a vast group of compounds known for their wide range of biological functions and health benefits. These include antioxidant and anti-inflammatory effects, along with antiviral, antibacterial, and antifungal properties. They also play a role in supporting immune function and exhibit anti-diabetic effects.

Polyphenols directly support the immune system and gut epithelium. In the microbiome, different polyphenols nourish different bacterial species—the greater the variety in your diet, the better. Some essential bacteria, like *Akkermansia*, don't survive without an adequate intake of these nutrients.

 The variety of colors in whole, plant-based meals enriches the variety of gut bacteria.

Certain polyphenols suppress bacterial growth. Typically, they are absorbed in the small intestine and don't reach the colon, leaving the microbiota crucial for colon health undisturbed. In the upper gut, they ensure a balanced microbiome by tackling *SIBO (Small Intestinal Bacterial Overgrowth)*, which we will cover in *Dimension 2*. Heat breaks down these compounds—another reason to enjoy an assortment of vegetables and fruits in their raw, dried, or frozen forms.

Some of the best sources of polyphenols include:

- Berries, grapes, and other colorful fruits
- Peppers, carrots, and artichokes
- Herbs and spices like cloves, peppermint, and star anise

- Nuts such as chestnuts and hazelnuts
- Flaxseed

Warning: Polyphenols, like *Resveratrol* and *Curcumin*, have become popular supplements. Approach them with caution—overconsumption can cause more harm than good, a problem more likely with pills than whole foods.

VITAMIN K

Vitamins play a crucial role in overall health. Many are obtained through your diet, but some, like Vitamin K in its K_2 form, are partly produced by your gut microbiota. A healthy microbiome can contribute up to half of your body's vitamin K needs. The other half must come from your diet. Studies show that while some bacteria make vitamin K, others consume it, making adequate intake important for your well-being and supporting a balanced microbial community. If your microbiome lacks variety, you may need to take a vitamin K supplement as your gut bacteria may not produce enough. This deficiency can lead to a self-perpetuating loop, where supplementing with vitamin K becomes essential to disrupt this pattern and reestablish a healthy balance.

The primary dietary source of vitamin K is green, leafy vegetables —best eaten raw. Since vitamin K is a fat-soluble vitamin, pairing leafy greens with olive or avocado oil in a salad improves its absorption. Supplements can be beneficial in the initial stages of healing, given that modern agricultural practices often deplete the natural vitamin content of fruits and vegetables. Should you opt for a supplement, pair vitamin K with vitamin D, as maintaining a balance between the two is essential. Generally, combining 50 μg/day of Vitamin K alongside 1000 IU of Vitamin D is considered safe for adults. However, consult with your healthcare provider before starting any new supplementation regimen.

See also:

- Key 2 ➢ Vitamin D

. . .

The Myth of Healthy Toppings on Junk Food

I often encounter a common misunderstanding about raw, bitter vegetables and other healthy eating habits with the people I coach. Many believe they can "fix" their junk food meals by tossing in a few healthy ingredients. It doesn't work that way. Adding a bit of onion to a pizza or sprinkling herbs on mac-n-cheese might boost the flavor, but it doesn't magically turn these meals into nutritious options. The underlying problem remains unaddressed: a heap of starch and processed dairy.

True transformation comes from seeing healthy food as a *replacement*, not just a *supplement*. It's about shifting from small doses of 'medicine' to full plates of nourishing meals.

 Healthy food is not a supplement to junk.

I advocate for a return to age-old eating habits—practiced for millennia in some cultures. Instead of grabbing a hot dog and fries with ketchup, a soft drink, and a cookie, try a piece of baked fish with a mixed salad of kale, onions, radishes, and other raw veggies dressed in olive oil and lemon juice or vinegar, seasoned with herbs and spices. If you find yourself longing for something sweet, consider dried fruits like dates or figs as a healthy dessert option. Drink a couple of glasses of water around 10-15 minutes BEFORE your meal (we will talk later about the right way to drink water). If you fancy something besides water, a bit of fruit juice or green tea before or a couple of hours after your meal works well—but skip the sweets and snacks.

You'll notice a shift in your taste preferences once you break the "addiction" to unhealthy foods and get on track with the active healing phase. Gradually, you'll begin to enjoy and genuinely prefer this healthier way of eating.

 Common doesn't equal normal.

It's easy to see why so many view autoimmune diseases as incurable. The key isn't just about changing what's on your plate but about transforming your entire lifestyle.

FOOD DIVERSITY

75% of the World's Food
Comes from 12 Plants and 5 Animal Species

Rank	Top Plants	Annual Global Production Metric Tons, 2011	Annual Global Value in USD Billions, 2012
1	Sugar	1,800,377,642	$57
2	Maize	885,289,935	$55
3	Rice	740,961,445	$337
4	Wheat	701,395,334	$84
5	Potatoes	373,158,351	$50
6	Soy Beans	262,037,569	$65
7	Cassava	256,404,044	$25
8	Tomatoes	159,347,031	$58
9	Banana	107,142,187	$29
10	Onions	86,343,822	$18
11	Apples	75,484,671	$32
12	Grapes	69,093,293	$39
Rank	Top Animals	Annual Global Production	Annual Global Value
1	Beef & Milk	725,123,869	$622
2	Chicken & Eggs	155,183,059	$182
3	Pork	118,168,709	$306
4	Goat Milk & Meat	20,000,000	n/a
5	Sheep	8,229,068	$22

Source: FAO via Wikipedia (http://bit.ly/2QAkmhC)

Appendix 1: Table 3.6 World food diversity. Source: https://thefuturemarket.com/biodiversity

Picture a vast cornfield stretching towards the horizon, offering plenty of food but supporting only a few animal species. Why? There's no lack of abundance, but unlike diverse grasslands, it's all the same type —corn. This leads to a dominance of certain animals adapted to this single food source, showing that ecosystem diversity relies on food variety, not just quantity.

Much like diverse grasslands support various species thanks to a range of foods, our gut bacteria also thrive on dietary variety. Each type of bacteria in your gut has a distinct reaction to the different foods you eat. A diet lacking in variety leads to a monotonous microbiome, much like our cornfield example. Remember, our goal is to nurture a microbiome that's more like a varied forest than a monoculture farm. Achieving this means including a wide range of foods in our diet.

It's a common misconception that variations in cooking methods mean a diverse diet. Whether fresh, sun-dried, canned, or made into a paste, a tomato is still a tomato. Though, the more it is processed from its fresh state, the less nutritious it becomes.

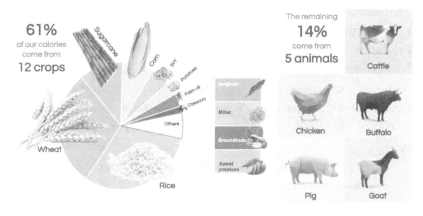

Appendix 1: Figure 3.7. Main crops and animals. The Food and Agriculture Organization (FAO) of the United Nations

Likewise, bread, pasta, pretzels, crackers, and wheat porridge all boil down to wheat—predominantly starch. In fact, many foods, from tortillas to potato chips, Tater Tots to various cereals and granolas, are primarily starch. Even whole-grain items like muesli or oatmeal are mostly starch, though they offer a richer palette of nutrients. Flour-based products are virtually all starch. As you can see, starch is possibly the most widespread ingredient in current diets, constituting roughly 60% of what a typical American consumes. Later, we'll explore the issues with a starch-heavy diet and how to avoid it; the focus now is on the need for food diversity.

Unfortunately, today, many people's microbiome resembles a monoculture cornfield. To improve your diet's diversity, be mindful while shopping and consider keeping a food diary. List the main ingredients of each meal—you might find that meals like pizza and mac-n-cheese, though seemingly different, are fundamentally the same, offering little beyond starch and cheese. This realization can be eye-opening, as the apparent variety in cooking methods masks the lack of nutritional diversity.

 It's the variety of raw whole food products that counts, not cooking styles.

Vegetarians and vegans can sometimes unintentionally limit their food spectrum even further. Yet, with thoughtful planning, a vegan diet can avoid this pitfall. With many more plant products available than animal-derived ones, expanding your selection of plant-based foods can compensate for the exclusion of animal products, ensuring a diet that's both diverse and supportive of a healthy microbiome.

Here's some food for thought in the form of startling statistics:

- 75% of our global food supply comes from just 12 plant and animal species.
- Half of our plant-based calories are sourced from just three staples: wheat, corn, and rice.
- Since 1900, there's been a 90% reduction in the variety of fruits and vegetables available in the US.

As agriculture has grown more industrialized, our diets have become less diverse. This pattern started early in human history, with agricultural societies consuming a smaller variety of foods than hunter-gatherers. The situation has further deteriorated recently as the market has become dominated by high-profit, low-risk products. Despite the existence of over 30,000 edible plants—some experts estimate up to 300,000—we consume only about 200 of them. The selection is even more restricted in a typical American supermarket, where you might find fewer than 40 kinds.

This limitation isn't just about plant species but also extends to the cultivars of each species. Economic viability often dictates what's available. There are about 7,500 apple varieties, 400 types of cabbage, and more than 150 types of pumpkin. But how many of these do you actually find in stores? A compelling illustration of this is the Cavendish banana's dominance in the marketplace, alongside maybe one or two other varieties, even though nature offers over 500 edible types of bananas.

We need a change in mindset. Welcome a diverse range of foods to your diet, and be open to trying new things whenever possible. Cuisines from regions like the Middle East, Central Asia, and India incorporate a broader range of plant species than many others. Step out of your regular grocery routine and try healthy ingredients from various ethnic cuisines. Online shopping, for example, breaks the boundaries of local availability. Expanding your culinary horizons means more than dining out. A local Mediterranean cafe will offer a broader menu than a fast-food chain. However, it still has a limited view of authentic Mediterranean cuisine, focusing only on popular and profitable items. Cooking at home allows you to explore a wider variety of dishes, as you're not constrained by the commercial motives that often limit restaurant menus. Experiment with different preparation methods and ingredient combinations. The aim is to eat more raw, whole plant foods, focusing on new ingredient combinations rather than just cooking techniques.

Remember, pathogenic bacteria feed on starch, sugar, and sweetened dairy. In contrast, a diet abundant in various raw vegetables supports a diverse microbiome, which is crucial for a robust immune system and overall health.

 Broaden the intrinsic diversity of your diet to cultivate a more diverse microbiome.

THE IMPORTANCE OF NATURAL CHILDBIRTH AND INFANT FEEDING

Even if it's too late for many, I am compelled to address this topic, as it can make a significant difference for the younger generation. Simply put, non-traditional childbirth and feeding methods may pose various risks to infants, including in the development of their immune systems.

The most critical milestones in forming a baby's microbiome and immunity happen at birth and in the following months. During natural childbirth, as the baby moves through the birth canal, they receive crucial microbiota from their mother. This process extends to breast-feeding, where the mother's microbiota further benefits the baby. Breast milk offers not only beneficial bacteria but also antibodies that inhibit the growth of harmful bacteria, laying a solid foundation for the baby's immune system. In contrast, many infant formulas and baby foods, sometimes containing ingredients like soy or sugars, fall short of replacing these natural probiotic and immune-boosting benefits.

While cesarean deliveries and baby formulas are necessary in specific situations for medical reasons, they should not be chosen solely for the sake of "convenience." In situations where they are unavoidable, focus on all other aspects to ensure a child's healthy microbiome and immunity development as soon as possible. This book offers strategies for these scenarios, but always consult a healthcare professional.

See also:
- Key 1 ➤ Sweet Does Not Equal Good
- Key 5 ➤ Xenoestrogens

CLIMATE AND MICROCLIMATE

Although our focus has been heavily on food and digestion, restoring an optimal microbiome composition calls for a more holistic approach. Elements such as outdoor time, exposure to everyday microbes, the use of hand sanitizers, and the microclimate of your home are all influential. I will cover these aspects in more detail in *Key 5*.

Before we proceed, let's take a closer look at the second microbiome dimension—*Distribution*. We'll come back to the *Composition* aspect later to explore more tactics.

See also:
- Key 5 ➤ The Hygiene Paradox: When Cleaning Backfires
- Key 5 ➤ Environment and Climate: Where You Live Matters

DIMENSION 2: MICROBIOME DISTRIBUTION

We've explored the "Who" of the microbiome; now let's focus on the equally important "Where." Bacterial concentration and diversity vary significantly across different parts of the gastrointestinal tract.

The stomach, despite regular exposure to germs in the food we eat, hosts very few bacteria. As we journey down the gastrointestinal tract, we observe increasing varieties and quantities of bacteria. The number quickly surpasses that of our own gut cells, growing denser as you approach the large intestine. The colon, the lowermost segment of the intestine, is a bustling metropolis of microorganisms, teeming with hundreds of billions of bacteria per gram of intestinal contents, home to approximately 1,000 species.

This uneven *Distribution* of bacteria in the human gut influences overall health and is tied to the *Microbiome Composition*. Any imbalance in this delicate setup can set off a domino effect, impacting multiple aspects of gut health. Fortunately, your body has several regulation mechanisms to maintain this balance.

See also:

• Appendix 1 ➢ Figure 3.8

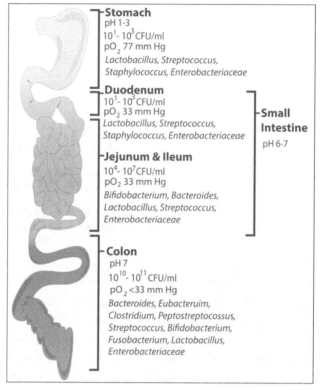

Stomach
pH 1-3
10^1- 10^3 CFU/ml
pO_2 77 mm Hg
Lactobacillus, Streptococcus,
Staphylococcus, Enterobacteriaceae

Duodenum
10^1- 10^3 CFU/ml
pO_2 33 mm Hg
Lactobacillus, Streptococcus,
Staphylococcus, Enterobacteriaceae

Jejunum & Ileum
10^4- 10^7 CFU/ml
pO_2 33 mm Hg
Bifidobacterium, Bacteroides,
Lactobacillus, Streptococcus,
Enterobacteriaceae

Small Intestine
pH 6-7

Colon
pH 7
10^{10}- 10^{11} CFU/ml
pO_2 <33 mm Hg
Bacteroides, Eubacteruim,
Clostridium, Peptostreptocossus,
Streptococcus, Bifidobacterium,
Fusobacterium, Lactobacillus,
Enterobacteriaceae

Appendix 1: Figure 3.8. Concentration of bacteria, oxygenation, and acidity across the digestive tract. Source: https://pharmrev. aspetjournals.org/content/71/2/198

KEY FACTORS FOR OPTIMAL MICROBIOME DISTRIBUTION

The human body employs various mechanisms to ensure the proper distribution of the gut microbiome. They include managing metabolic microniches, maintaining pH levels, dynamic microbe-tissue interactions, and regulating oxygen concentration.

In this book, I discuss the following key factors that support and enhance these natural mechanisms:

1. Food ingredients and eating habits.
2. Stomach acid.
3. Bile.

4. Overall healthy digestion: This includes everything from chewing and salivating to the role of digestive juices.

5. Healthy gut epithelium: This involves how the cells lining your intestine interact with bacteria, encouraging some while controlling or eliminating others. The epithelium repair is covered in *Key 3. Leaky Gut: Repair.*

6. Healthy gut motility: Essential for preventing bacterial overgrowth in localized areas by actively moving digestive contents consistently in a single direction. Normalizing motility is addressed in *Key 4. Lazy Gut: Reawaken.*

7. Oral microbiome health: Often overlooked, this is the second most crucial microbiome in the human body, as it constantly sends migrating microbes down to your digestive tract. This is covered in the *Eliminate Other Autoimmune Triggers* chapter in *Key 5.*

We'll cover points 1 to 4 in more detail in this *Key 1* section of the book.

CONSEQUENCES OF WRONG MICROBIOME DISTRIBUTION

The microbiome's distribution can sometimes become disrupted, even with the numerous regulatory mechanisms. This imbalance often leads to an overabundance of bacteria in early segments of the digestive tract, like the stomach and upper intestines, triggering a series of issues.

Bacteria that increase in these areas can absorb significant amounts of nutrients as they multiply, affecting both your health and the beneficial microbiome further downstream. They also interfere with normal digestion by harming the gut epithelium and altering the environment's chemistry. Additionally, these microbes produce toxins during food fermentation, causing a range of issues, from irritating and damaging the gut cells to overburdening the liver with a toxic load. Depending on the severity of the problem, this chronic poisoning can have extensive effects on the entire body, including the brain. Consequently, both you and your lower gut microbiome end up with more toxins and fewer nutrients.

This changes the whole gut ecosystem. The colon and lower intestine microbiota are robbed of their nutrients, and the toxins released by the excessive bacteria upstream harm the beneficial bacteria, reducing their numbers and diversity. In such conditions, many beneficial bacteria struggle to thrive, often leading to the survival of only the most aggressive strains. This negatively affects the quantity and variety of the microbiome, further aggravating the imbalance and causing the *Microbiome Composition* to shift in an unfavorable direction.

This pathological microbial growth directly impacts the immune system within the gut, leading to chronic inflammation that exhausts the entire immune system. This can result in issues like allergies, autoimmune diseases, and a weakened immune response. Over time, it might even increase the risk of cancer development.

The most noticeable manifestation of this kind of skewed *Microbiome Distribution* is what's known as SIBO, or *Small Intestinal Bacterial Overgrowth*.

THE MANY FACES OF MICROBIOME MALDISTRIBUTION: SIBO, IBS, IBD, AND ULCERS

SMALL INTESTINAL BACTERIAL OVERGROWTH (SIBO)

You may have heard of SIBO from your healthcare provider, particularly if gut-related symptoms have become severe enough to need attention. It stands for *Small Intestinal Bacterial Overgrowth* and involves an abnormal increase in bacteria—usually the unhealthy kind—in the upper part of the small intestine. We went over the mechanisms and consequences of SIBO in the previous chapter.

Let's take it a step further. My concept of *Disrupted Microbiome Distribution* covers more than just the small intestine. It also includes harmful stomach bacteria, changes in the oral microbiome, and issues in the colon microbiome. It's all connected. I'm introducing this broader term to highlight that:

 Microbiome Distribution and Microbiome Composition are two interconnected, synergistic aspects of the microbiome that can be disrupted and should be addressed in tandem.

SIBO SYMPTOMS

While SIBO initially affects the gut, its effects often go beyond the gastrointestinal (GI) system. Some of these include:

- Abdominal pain, particularly after meals
- Bloating and abdominal distension
- Cramps and indigestion (dyspepsia)
- Constant feeling of fullness
- Gas, flatulence, and mucus in stool
- Constipation or chronic diarrhea/loose stools
- Increased bloating after consuming carbs, fiber, and sugar
- Nausea and vomiting
- Foul-smelling, sticky stools
- Unintentional weight loss, despite supplement use
- Anemia
- Nutrient malabsorption, including iron and other minerals
- Vitamin deficiencies, such as B_{12}, K
- Fatigue, depression, and neurological issues
- Bone density reduction

BELOW THE WATERLINE: SUBCLINICAL SIBO

When medically diagnosed, various previously mentioned symptoms can point to a disrupted microbiome distribution, including SIBO. Unfortunately, a substantial number of cases go undetected.

Studies suggest that 13% to 35% of seemingly healthy individuals may have subclinical, symptomless SIBO, with people experiencing discomfort only in certain situations. In other words, up to a third of the population is likely mildly affected by this condition, not seriously enough for diagnosis and treatment, but it still lingers below the waterline. This underlying issue can gradually undermine the intricate balance between the microbiome, gut, and immune system. Over time, the resulting imbalance can compromise the immune system, potentially leading to autoimmune diseases.

For years, some might experience mild fleeting symptoms. For instance, many people feel bloated after eating prebiotic foods like cabbage, onions, or legumes; or probiotic foods such as naturally fermented sauerkraut. This is due to an imbalance in the *microbiota distribution*. In a healthy gut, these foods don't cause bloating, cramps, or gas. Instead of tackling the root cause, people often choose to avoid eating large quantities of raw vegetables, essentially sweeping the issue under the rug. This is like hiding dumbbells to conceal muscle weakness. You can live with this condition for years by avoiding things that trigger symptoms. Yet, even the low-level chronic inflammation caused by subclinical SIBO can, in the long run, lead to severe health problems, including autoimmune diseases or even cancer.

See also:
• Diseases Related to Immune System Disorders

Irritable Bowel Syndrome (IBS)

SIBO and *Irritable Bowel Syndrome* (IBS) often go hand in hand, with abnormal microbiome distribution potentially leading to irritation and damage to the gut epithelium. The symptoms of IBS are similar to SIBO, including:

- Abdominal pain, cramping, or bloating
- Diarrhea, constipation, or a mix of both
- Changes in bowel movement frequency and appearance
- Flatulence and excess gas
- Mucus in the stool, often appearing whitish

- Urgent need to go to the bathroom
- A feeling of incomplete evacuation after defecation
- Food sensitivities, stress, or hormonal changes
- Unexplained vomiting
- Weight loss
- Iron deficiency anemia

SIBO and IBS often fly under the radar for years. If you've been diagnosed with one of these conditions, it's probably because your symptoms became too severe to ignore. It's believed that around 10-15% of adults in the US might be part of this not-so-exclusive club.

Constant irritation in the gut isn't just a minor annoyance—it can escalate, leading to more severe conditions like *Inflammatory Bowel Disease (IBD): Ulcerative Colitis* and *Crohn's Disease*. In this way, IBS can be seen as a potential precursor to more severe illnesses. Chronic irritation also stresses and exhausts immune cells, potentially leading to issues in the immune system. Studies have shown that IBS is a risk factor for a range of other conditions, including *scleroderma, arthritis, lupus,* other autoimmune disorders, *allergies,* and, surprisingly, *diabetes* and *Parkinson's* disease.

This underscores the importance of addressing microbiome distribution and gut lining health. The *5R+ System* is designed to target these issues, improving immune health. For more on repairing the gut epithelium, see *Key 3.*

ULCERS AND HELICOBACTER PYLORI

In a bold move back in 1984, Australian Dr. Barry Marshall embarked on a risky experiment with the only human subject he could legally use—himself. He ingested a solution containing *Helicobacter pylori*, a recently discovered bacterium, to prove its role in causing stomach and duodenal ulcers. His experiment was a success, albeit a risky one. Luckily, Marshall treated himself effectively and later recounted this adventurous tale while accepting his Nobel Prize. The well-known ulcer disease, which often requires serious surgery, is caused by the same issue we've been exploring: *Disrupted Microbiome*

Distribution and *Composition*. As mentioned previously, the stomach and the initial part of the small intestine should have an almost non-existent bacterial presence. Yet, recent studies show that about 50% to 75% of people today have *Helicobacter pylori* in their stomachs, though often without noticeable symptoms—a situation similar to the subclinical SIBO and IBS we've discussed. Indeed, a disrupted microbiome can manifest in various ways.

COMMON APPROACHES TO SIBO AND WHY THEY ARE DANGEROUS

There are several tactics for tackling SIBO or, more broadly, the improper distribution of microbiota. Below, I discuss three frequently used methods that, despite their popularity, can lead to adverse side effects, especially with long-term use. Beyond these, there exist natural and safe approaches to managing SIBO, which we will explore in the upcoming chapter.

Disclaimer: If your doctor has recommended any of the methods mentioned below, they might have specific reasons based on your health situation. It's advisable to discuss any concerns with your healthcare provider or consider a second opinion from another medical professional if necessary. Always consult your doctor before implementing any strategies mentioned in this book.

See also:

• Key 1 ➤ Healthy Digestion to Fix Microbiota Distribution

KILL'EM ALL: ANTIBIOTICS

Faced with excess bacteria, it might seem logical to turn to antibiotics and attempt a 'kill 'em all' approach. Right? Wrong! This method is flawed because antibiotics don't discriminate; they wipe out beneficial bacteria—vital for your gut health—along with the harmful ones. This approach creates a population vacuum, quickly filled by resistant, more aggressive strains, including fungi. So, instead of resolving one issue, you end up with multiple new problems.

The key to reshaping the microbiota lies in transforming the entire ecosystem, which is the central aim of this holistic *5R+ System*. Unfortunately, despite these drawbacks, antibiotics continue to be a go-to solution for treating SIBO symptoms, even with the known risks of further disrupting the microbiome.

FLUSH IT DOWN

A standard no-drug recommendation for mitigating the problem is to drink more water with food. This approach may reduce irritation and inflammation as it flushes out bacteria and toxins, preventing their accumulation in one place. Yet, it is terrible for digestion. It also does not tackle the underlying cause of SIBO. Instead, digestive juices are diluted, impairing their ability to break down food and regulate gut microbiota properly. This leads to partially digested food and harmful bacteria being transported to other parts of the gastrointestinal tract, potentially damaging the epithelium downstream.

The following chapter explores the importance of maintaining proper stomach acid and bile concentration. In Key 4, we will also cover more about hydration principles. Here's a quick rule of thumb:

 Drink water before and between meals, but not during or immediately after eating.

Habitual flushing is a band-aid solution, showing that even non-medication strategies can backfire on your health. Essentially, it's a misguided attempt to compensate for reduced *Intestinal Motility*. Under normal conditions, food should steadily progress through the digestive system as it breaks down, neither too fast nor too slow. Too fast will disrupt digestion; too slow creates stagnation and bacterial build-up. Normalizing Motility is an essential focus of the 5R+ System and is thoroughly discussed in *Key 4*.

See also:
• Key 1 ➢ Healthy Digestion to Fix Microbiota Distribution
• Key 4 ➢ Water: Drink Right

STARVE THEM: LOW-FODMAP DIET

I've seen many people with *Rheumatoid Arthritis* (RA) and *Crohn's disease* who have all but given up on vegetables, especially raw ones, fearing they would stir up bowel troubles or RA flare-ups. However, avoiding veggies doesn't extinguish small intestinal bacterial over-growth (SIBO); it just keeps it simmering undetected like coals under ashes, ready to flare up at any time. This 'out of sight, out of mind' tactic gradually undermines immune and digestive health. You need to address the root of the problem, which includes getting rid of SIBO rather than keeping it in hibernation.

This is the issue with the *low-FODMAP diet*—often the go-to solu-tion for reducing abnormal bacterial growth caused by improper microbiome distribution. It involves eliminating various bacteria-feeding foods from your diet, effectively starving the pathogenic popu-lation. However, this strategy also inadvertently deprives the beneficial microbiota of nutrients, particularly those in the colon, where a high concentration of bacteria is vital.

By minimizing prebiotics essential for a healthy microbiome, the *low-FODMAP diet* reduces the variety of foods and nutrients you consume, leading to fiber deficiency. Fiber is necessary for healthy motility and the production of gut-nourishing *short-chain fatty acids (SCFAs)*—an indispensable source of energy for the intestinal epithe-lium. We will cover more on SCFAs in *Key 3*.

> Starving the microbiota inevitably starves the gut epithelium.

Even though many versions of the low-FODMAP diet try to address these issues by striking a balance, they all tend to be unnatural and unhealthy. They're far from what we'd consider regular, everyday whole food. These diets focus more on managing symptoms than tack-ling the root cause. In contrast, the 5R+ System is designed to nurture a healthy microbial and digestive ecosystem. It aims to naturally prevent the overgrowth of harmful bacteria and ensure their proper distribu-tion by leveraging ecological niches.

While low-FODMAP diets might offer a quick fix, they increase the risk of long-term complications. If your doctor recommends this diet, consider it a temporary stopgap while working on broader health goals. It's like strategically pulling back in one area to make gains elsewhere, setting the stage for a successful counterattack. This approach exemplifies the synergy between different strategies within the 5R+ program. Ideally, you should aim to switch to a diet rich in various raw, whole-plant foods packed with prebiotics as soon as possible. However, ramping up your prebiotic intake should be paired with improvements in *gut motility* as described in *Key 4*.

See also:

• Key 3 ➤ Nutrition For the Gut Epithelium

NAVIGATING THE MINEFIELD

Tackling severe SIBO can be challenging, but the positive outcomes are worth the effort. It often requires a careful blend of various 5R+ strategies applied methodically and thoughtfully. Beyond improving motility, acid, bile, and digestive juices, it's worth incorporating herbs and spices that help control bacterial growth. Techniques like meal spacing, water-fasting, and specific gut-flushing exercises can also help. The next chapter focuses on broader strategies for managing *Microbiome Distribution*, including SIBO.

The goal is to smoothly transition from a low-FODMAP diet to a diverse diet rich in raw, whole-plant foods and probiotics. For those grappling with more severe IBS/SIBO conditions, this may mean longer periods of water-fasting and significant enhancements in gut motility before you can safely increase prebiotic and probiotic intake— and even then, be careful. This is why it's essential to work on other areas simultaneously, significantly improving *Motility (Key 4)* and reducing *Inflammation (Key 2)* while also employing the strategies covered in the following chapter.

HEALTHY DIGESTION TO FIX MICROBIOTA DISTRIBUTION

In the previous chapter, we looked at various popular methods for addressing SIBO, which are often as ineffective as sweeping dust under the rug. For better results, I recommend shifting your focus towards rebuilding your body's primary natural mechanisms for controlling *Microbiome Distribution*, starting with improving digestion. Poor digestion and SIBO often go hand-in-hand, feeding off each other and worsening the situation.

The following factors for managing your microbiota distribution directly through digestive health address the root cause of the problem:

- Normal activity of digestive juices.
- Acid.
- Bile.
- Mastication and salivation.
- Active gastrointestinal motility.
- Frequency of meals.
- Eat more foods that regulate microbiota balance.
- Avoid foods that trigger harmful microbial growth.

In the following chapters, we will go through these factors step by step.

Food naturally introduces a vast range of bacteria into our bodies. Limiting their survival helps maintain a balanced gut microbiome. By focusing on the abovementioned factors, you can cultivate a digestive environment where very few of these incoming bacteria can settle. With fewer "immigrants" your body maintains better control. This approach allows your microbiome to develop in a way that's more aligned with your body's natural regulatory processes, ensuring a healthier gut ecosystem.

DON'T RUSH THE REACTOR

Think of digestion as a chemical reactor where food mixes with digestive juices—your body's chemical agents. To ensure this reaction runs smoothly, several key factors are essential:

- **Concentration**: High-quality and the right amount of chemical reagents—digestive juices.
- **Mix**: Finer food particles blend more effectively with the reagents and dissolve more quickly.
- **Time:** Sufficient time for the reaction to occur.

We'll talk about enhancing your digestive juices shortly. For now, remember it's crucial to avoid diluting them. Like in any chemical reaction, diluting the reactants—making them less concentrated or washing them away too soon—impairs the process. This happens when you drink water with or right after your meals. Doing so weakens the activity of digestive juices and accelerates the movement of incompletely digested food through the gut. While hydration is essential, timing is everything. Keep water separate from meals to let the digestive juices do their job undisturbed.

For a similar reason, thorough mastication (chewing) is essential. The finer the food particles, the better they mix with the reagents, speeding up digestion. At every step, food should be thoroughly processed by secreted digestive juices. This prevents abnormal bacterial growth in the stomach and the first part of the intestine. These bacteria feast on improperly digested food, hijacking your nutrients and producing unwanted toxins. When you introduce food into your personal "chemical reactor," remember: bacteria are competing with you for those nutrients.

 Do not sabotage your digestion.

Another reason not to rush the reactor is that large molecules (macromolecules) must be efficiently broken down into their smallest components (monomers) before moving further along the digestive tract. Doing so prevents partially digested food from passing through the gut lining, triggering the immune response and causing inflammation. The less time those macromolecules hang around, the better. We will talk about this in more detail in *Key 3*. If food is not effectively fermented, indicating poor digestion, it can fuel both SIBO and inflammation. Factors potentially contributing to this problem include:

- Dumping—food moving through the stomach too fast.
- Not chewing food thoroughly.
- Poor quality of diluted digestive juices.

As you work on *Key 3* to heal your epithelium, its function will improve, and you'll notice better digestion.

In the following chapters, we will explore all these aspects in detail, along with other key strategies for optimal gut health, including mastication and two essential chemical reagents in your toolkit: *acid* and *bile*.

See also:
- Key 4 ➤ Water: Drink Right
- Key 3 ➤ Obstacle #9: Chilled Food and Drinks

DUMPING

In most cases, food moves through the stomach too quickly due to:

- The consumption of cold items, like ice cream or chilled drinks, which will be covered in *Key 3*.

- Surgical procedures that remove a significant portion of the stomach.

See also:
- Key 3 ➤ Eliminate Obstacles ➤ Obstacle #9: Chilled Food and Drinks

SURGICAL PROCEDURES TO AVOID

Dumping syndrome commonly occurs after the stomach is partially or completely removed. The procedure results in food bypassing crucial digestive steps that usually occur in the stomach, leading to undigested food moving rapidly through the intestines. Such a procedure is necessary for conditions like tumors. Unfortunately, it is increasingly used to combat obesity through what's known as *bariatric surgery*. Though offering quick results, it can lead to a range of health problems, jeopardizing both digestive and immune system functions. In solving one problem, it creates others, turning weight loss—the visible result—into a misleading sign of success.

Lifestyle changes are the best way to tackle obesity. Although targeting immune health, following the nutritional principles in the 5R+ System will help normalize your weight. Choosing to remove an essential, functioning organ to address a condition better managed through lifestyle changes is a highly questionable approach.

MASTICATION AND SALIVATION – THE UNDERRATED DUO

Chewing (mastication) and saliva are important for microbiome and gut lining health, a topic we will cover in more detail in *Key 3*. Thorough mastication breaks down your food into smaller particles, making it easier to blend with digestive enzymes for quicker digestion. Conversely, larger food pieces take longer to digest and absorb, giving bacteria in the initial part of the small intestine a source of nutrients.

Additionally, stomach acid doesn't effectively infiltrate these bigger particles, allowing any harmful bacteria inside them to survive and be smuggled through the stomach into the intestine. Such microbes can only be eliminated in food that has been thoroughly chewed and mixed with stomach acid. As discussed, minimizing these "immigration waves" of bacteria is vital to avoid disrupting *Microbiome Distribution*.

It is important that saliva is mixed with your food when you chew. It has antibacterial and fermentative properties, kickstarting the digestive process. Compromising this initial digestive step means putting extra strain on your stomach and the initial section of your intestine.

See more:

• Key 3 ➤ Obstacle #7: Insufficient Mastication
• Key 4 ➤ Physical Activities for Optimal Bowel Transit ➤ Chewing

STOMACH ACID

Acid — The Protective Firewall

Stomach acid has several functions, from helping digest proteins to defending against infections and the overgrowth of unwanted bacteria. As the body's first protective firewall, stomach acid effectively destroys harmful bacteria present in our food.

It's estimated that between 22% and 50% of people have low stomach acid levels, a condition known as *hypochlorhydria*. This allows bacteria from food to flourish in the first part of the intestine, and sometimes even in the stomach. What's meant to be a protective shield becomes a breeding ground for harmful microbes, leading to issues such as *gastritis* and *ulcers*. It can also cause so-called *heartburn* (*gastroesophageal reflux*), which I will return to later. The impact of an imbalanced microbiome distribution is far-reaching, also causing conditions like SIBO, which can weaken the immune system, and *hypoacid gastritis*, increasing the risk of stomach cancer. Often, these issues can fly under the radar for a long time.

That's precisely why tactics to maintain the right level of stomach acidity are a cornerstone of the 5R+ System—keeping your internal protective firewall alert and active.

DILUTION OF DIGESTIVE JUICES

Digestive juices are often inadvertently diluted when you drink during meals, washing away stomach acid and speeding up the passage of food through the digestive system. As a result, the acid and enzymes may not kill all the bacteria, and partially digested food may travel downstream, irritating the intestinal epithelium. Liquid meals like soups, which mix a small amount of solid food with a lot of water, present a similar challenge. With few exceptions, opting for solid, well-chewed food over more watery alternatives is better. This principle extends to all digestive juices: they must be undiluted to work effectively.

Your body needs a significant amount of water, and water is necessary for proper digestion, but timing is everything. Drink water before and between meals, not with or directly after. Rather, let food and stomach juices mingle undisturbed without the company of drinks. Wait 15 minutes after drinking water before eating, and 1 to 3 hours after eating before drinking again, depending on your meal—less time for fruits and more for protein-rich foods, especially meat.

Avoid chilled drinks during or shortly after meals as they can abnormally stimulate motility, leading to the stomach "dumping" food prematurely, resulting in incomplete digestion. Additionally, the cold can negatively impact the stomach's epithelial cells, reducing digestive juice production. The habit of drinking with meals is particularly damaging if the beverages are high in sugar or artificially sweetened.

See also:

• Key 3 ➤ Eliminate Obstacles ➤ Obstacle #9: Chilled Food and Drinks

• Key 4 ➤ Water: Drink Right

WHAT CAUSES LOW STOMACH ACID

Several factors can lead to reduced stomach acid production:

- Aging (I know, there's nothing we can do about it).
- High sugar diets.
- High starch diets.
- Poor protein intake.
- Low Zinc or Iron status.
- Deficiency in B_1 and other B vitamins.
- Chronic stress.
- Insufficient mastication or eating on the run.
- Antacid medications like proton pump inhibitors and H_2 blockers, including over-the-counter options.
- *Helicobacter pylori* bacteria.

Addressing these factors helps maintain healthy stomach acid levels. I cover most of these topics in other chapters.

Take note that efficient chewing not only prepares food for digestion but also stimulates the production of all digestive juices—gastric acid included.

IMPROVE STOMACH JUICE PRODUCTION

Besides managing the negative factors that reduce stomach acid, there are several steps you can take to actively stimulate acid production. Integrating these habits into your daily life can help normalize your gastric acidity levels:

- Thorough and active food mastication.
- Consuming foods that stimulate healthy acid production, such as:
  - Bitter vegetables.
  - Fermented vegetables and pickles.
  - Spices and herbs.
  - Adding acidic foods, like lemon, lime, vinegar, tamarind, tart cherries, Cornelian cherry, sour plums (aloo-Bukhara, alcha), pomegranate, etc., to your meals.

Bitter vegetables, spices, and herbs have been staples in diets for thousands of years, meaning their safety is time-tested. Similarly, pickles, including those available in supermarkets that might not be genuinely fermented, can enhance acid production. The importance of these food groups is discussed throughout this book as they offer multiple benefits in the 5R+ system.

Finally, introducing a small amount of acid to your meals is a tasty way to support stomach acidity. Sprinkle your food with lemon or lime, whether whole or as juice, or add vinegar to help counterbalance insufficient acid production in the stomach and promote proper digestion.

All these meal additions are even more essential with protein-rich foods. Proteins require more acid for optimal digestion and pose a higher risk of inflammatory reactions if not completely digested quickly.

See more:

- Key 1 ➤ Actively Repopulate ➤ Feeding your Allies ➤ Good Bitter Truth

NATURAL SUPPLEMENTS — APPROACH WITH CAUTION

Some unconventional ingredients can also improve the quality of stomach juices and aid digestion. While these ingredients aren't typically found in everyday diets, they're generally safe for short-term use. However, be mindful of dosages and consult with your healthcare provider before trying these:

- Aloe vera.
- Artichoke leaf.
- Hops.
- Dandelion.
- Gentian.

Products marketed as "Digestive Bitters" feature a mix of different bitter plant extracts that can also help digestion.

Warning: Pregnant or breastfeeding women should avoid most digestive bitters, particularly those containing *gentian, burdock, Aloe* *vera*, and *angelica*.

I mention these supplements because they are well-known, and you may have seen them recommended. Still, focusing on healthy diet and lifestyle changes, along with the safe foods previously discussed, is a much more sustainable approach than relying on such supplements.

Antacids and "Heartburn" (Gastroesophageal Reflux)

Antacids, often used to alleviate "heartburn," are one of the most frequent causes of low stomach acid. "Heartburn," more accurately termed *gastroesophageal reflux*, happens when acidic stomach contents flow back up, irritating the *esophagus*—the part of the digestive tract that connects your throat to your stomach. It's easy to understand why many mistakenly think stomach acid is the villain in this story. However, stomach acid is essential for digestion and overall well-being. Low levels can lead to issues like small intestinal bacterial overgrowth (SIBO), immune system problems, and even stomach cancer. Under normal circumstances, stomach contents do not reflux upwards; healthy motility ensures everything moves in one direction only—downwards. Also, the stomach's entrance seals shut, preventing any contact between stomach acid and the esophagus.

Treating gastroesophageal reflux with antacids isn't effective. The underlying problem isn't too much acid but rather issues with poor motility and/or bacteria in the stomach. Interestingly, many patients already have low stomach acid, and it often contributes to this condition. As previously mentioned, food isn't effectively digested when acid levels are low, allowing bacteria to flourish in the stomach. This increases bacterial fermentation and gas, creating pressure that forces stomach contents upward in reflux. Hence, "heartburn" can result from improper *Microbiome Distribution*, something the 5R+ System seeks to correct.

It's crucial to determine the cause of your heartburn. If your stomach acid level is already low, antacids might make things worse. Always talk to a healthcare professional who can help you identify the problem—boosting your stomach acid might be the right solution.

While this book doesn't focus extensively on gastroesophageal reflux, here are a few tips to help you navigate this challenge as you work on resolving the DILL+ locks.

First, addressing *Dysbiosis* and enhancing *Motility* (covered in *Keys 1* and *4*) can often alleviate the problem. Adjusting microbiome distribution eliminates bacterial overgrowth and prevents the formation of excessive gas and pressure in the stomach that lead to reflux issues. Additionally, strengthening weak digestive tract motility muscles ensures active one-directional food movements, preventing backflow. Finally, these muscles tightly close the stomach entrance, blocking the escape of stomach contents back up into the esophagus.

Another simple yet effective tip is to eat smaller meals to decrease food volume and pressure in the stomach. I also recommend not eating anything 4 hours before bedtime. Keeping upright when your stomach is full helps prevent upward reflux. Since the muscles sealing your stomach's entrance tend to relax during sleep, going to bed with an empty stomach can minimize reflux and give your digestive system a break—we'll touch on this again in *Key 3*.

While antacids may offer quick relief from "heartburn," they don't tackle the root cause of the problem. They might even worsen it by promoting bacterial growth in the stomach and small intestine. These bacteria and their toxins can lead to inflammation, negatively affecting stomach muscles and motility function. I encourage you to speak with your doctor to uncover the real issue. It's often more effective to reduce the use of antacid medication and focus on addressing the underlying cause instead.

Adverse Effect of a Low Protein Diet

A diet low in protein reduces the production of stomach juices, including acid, which are essential for digestion. People following a vegan or vegetarian lifestyle often encounter this issue, as their diet might not include sufficient protein-rich foods. Remember, opting for a vegan or vegetarian path doesn't automatically equate to healthier eating. I've observed quite a few people who've gone vegetarian only to end up eating less nutritious food. In fact, a diet high in starch, sugar, and trans-fats can be entirely vegan yet a sure path to a hospital bed.

 Vegan does not automatically mean healthy.

However, if done right, a vegan or vegetarian diet can indeed be very healthy, even superior to diets that include animal products. The key is to balance your nutrients well, avoid vegan junk food, and fill your plate with a variety of whole, raw, plant-based foods. Also, ensure you eat enough protein in the form of lentils, beans, seeds, and nuts. If you have sensitivities, be cautious with nuts, as they can trigger inflammation.

In general, all high-protein foods may cause inflammation. We will return to this topic in *Key 3*. As you progress through the DILL+ locks, inflammatory responses should subside, enabling you to gradually add more protein-rich products to your plate.

See also:

• Key 3 ➤ Proteins and Animal Products

BILE AND LIVER HEALTH

The effectiveness of stomach acid rapidly decreases once it moves out of the stomach, but that's where another factor comes into play: *bile*. Produced by the liver, it maintains a hostile environment for pathogens and regulates bacterial growth in the intestine.

Bile, a mix of acids and salts, is essential for fat digestion and vitamin absorption. It also partners with stomach acid to influence the gut microbiome's ecosystem. Disrupted microbiota in both the small and large intestines can often be linked to insufficient levels of bile acids, known for their antimicrobial properties.

Effective elimination of waste also depends on bile acids. Low levels can slow the breakdown of metabolic waste, possibly leading to constipation and flatulence, symptoms frequently associated with *IBS-C (Irritable Bowel Syndrome with Constipation)*. In *Lazy Gut* scenarios, constipation can sometimes be interrupted by brief periods of diarrhea triggered by changes in diet, like eating fatty meals. Addressing bile deficiencies and improving bile quality can improve chemical balance and the gut microbiota as well as alleviate these Lazy Gut symptoms.

BILE SALT MALABSORPTION AND THE MICROBIOME

Some people choose to avoid oils and foods that stimulate bile production because they have *bile salt malabsorption (BSMA)*, another condition closely linked to *Dysbiosis*. But, on a hopeful note: repopulating your microbiome can improve this condition.

Bile isn't just for digestion; it's crucial for nutrient absorption and regulating your microbiome. These functions require many chemical transformations of bile, driven by gut bacteria activity. In a healthy digestive tract, beneficial bacteria transform bile compounds, boosting their diversity and enhancing their function. These altered bile salts are later reabsorbed in the lower part of the small intestine and returned to the liver—the body's chemical factory—for reuse. It's fascinating how a healthy microbiome powers your bodily functions, including defense against harmful guests. However, when dysbiosis—microbial imbalance—strikes, this process can malfunction, leading to poor digestion, inflammation, and altered liver metabolism, often resulting in *IBS-D* (*Irritable Bowel Syndrome with Diarrhea*).

> N-3 oils, also known as Omega-3 fatty acids, are essential fats that our bodies need but can't produce. Found in fish oil and plant-based foods such as flaxseeds, chia seeds, walnuts, and pecans, these fats must be included in your diet to support overall well-being.

Research continues to unfold, but it's clear that microbiome health, inflammation levels, and bile-related issues are all closely linked. Addressing these factors **simultaneously** is crucial for your well-being. If you're dealing with bile salt malabsorption or fat-triggered diarrhea, reducing fat intake might bring some relief. But there's more you can do. Adopt 5R+ tactics, focus on beneficial N-3 oils in moderation, and increase fiber intake to improve microbiome and liver health.

As always, seek personalized guidance from your healthcare provider.

See also:
- Key 2 ➤ Fats and Oils
- Key 4 ➤ Your Food and Gut Motility

THE ESSENTIALS OF HEALTHY BILE PRODUCTION

The functions of the liver, one of the largest and most complex organs in your body, include digestion, blood purification, metabolism, and detoxification. It can be compared to a central chemical lab or factory churning out essential substances. Among the liver's many "product lines" is bile, which is necessary for intestinal and microbiome health.

If you are struggling with bile deficiency, possibly due to liver or gallbladder conditions, or if you had your gallbladder removed, *bile salt supplements* can offer a much-needed boost, compensating for the reduced natural production. These supplements are widely accessible without prescription and are typically well-tolerated. Of course, always consult your healthcare professional before starting any supplement regimen, especially if you're managing other health issues.

Even without specific liver or gallbladder problems, you can naturally enhance your bile quality and production by adjusting your lifestyle and diet. Here's how you can do it:

- **Hydration:** This is non-negotiable for your liver's detox and bile production. As previously mentioned, aim to drink plenty of water between meals, not during or right after them.
- **Weight management:** If you carry extra weight, even a slight reduction can significantly boost your liver health and bile production.
- **Maintaining liver health:** Reducing the liver's toxic load is crucial. We'll explore this topic further below.
- **Diet:** Focus on foods that stimulate bile production and enhance liver health, including:

- Healthy oils
- Bitter vegetables and herbs
- *Hepatoprotective* foods and other nutrients for liver health.

In this chapter, we'll walk through practical, everyday tactics to support your liver, encourage healthy bile production, and help your digestive system run smoothly.

See also:

• Key 4 ➤ Water: Drink Right

HELPING YOUR LIVER

REDUCE TOXIC LOAD

Among its many functions, your liver works tirelessly to detoxify your body and neutralize toxins from what you eat and the environment. But, if your diet is loaded with toxins, it can overwhelm this vital organ, hampering its function. In the worst-case scenario, this toxic overload can lead to the accumulation of toxins within the liver tissue, causing liver cell damage. However, there's good news!

> **The liver restores remarkably well; just stop poisoning it.**

You have the power to lighten this burden. By making mindful choices to reduce the intake of toxins, you can help your liver heal and regain its efficiency. This will boost bile production while ensuring your liver stays on top of its game as the central chemical hub of your body.

Here's how you can reduce the toxic load on your liver:

- Say no to alcohol!
- Avoid hydrogenated oils (including trans-fats) and artificial food additives

- Eat less meat
- Choose organic foods
- Boost your diet with fiber and raw vegetables
- Promote proper gut motility (see *Key 4*)
- Restore healthy microbiota (*Key 1*)

Alcohol is a potent toxin that strains the liver's detox abilities. New research shows it also alters the microbiome and increases gut permeability. While alcohol consumption may be deeply ingrained in many cultures, I strongly advise avoiding this toxin.

Hydrogenated oils and artificial food additives aren't doing your liver any favors, either. We'll cover more about this topic soon.

Every time we eat, our intestines produce toxins, and it's the liver's job to clean them up. Meat digestion, specifically, is like a heavy lifting session for your liver, loading it up with toxins. Therefore, cutting back on meat gives your liver a much-needed break to heal and restore. Conversely, vegetables are easier on your liver and don't produce as many toxins when broken down. So, even if you're not vegan, cutting back on meat and ramping up plant-based foods can be a game-changer for your liver's health.

 Even for non-vegetarians, meat should not be an everyday food.

Maintaining optimal digestive motility is crucial for removing toxic waste quickly from your gut, which, in turn, eases the workload on your liver. Additionally, restoring a healthy gut microbiota will reduce the production of harmful toxins. That's where a diet rich in dietary fiber and raw vegetables comes into play. Think of fiber as a natural cleanup crew, swiftly escorting toxins out of your system.

By filling your diet with fiber-rich foods, you enhance the elimination of toxins and reduce the amount produced during digestion, particularly if you add raw vegetables to the mix. Consuming meat occasionally is possible with this kind of diet. But if your meals are predominately starch-based, adding meat can amplify issues. It increases toxin production and contributes to a *Lazy gut* and disrupted microbiome, piling on more toxins for your liver and gut epithelium to deal with. We will return to this in *Key 3*.

 Give your liver and gut adequate time to restore.

See also:
- Key 2 ➤ Fats and Oils
- Key 1 ➤ Chemical Additives and Toxins in Our Food
- Key 4 ➤ The Fiber Paradox: Why Eat What You Can't Digest
- Key 3 ➤ Obstacle #3: Toxic Byproducts of Digestion

HEPATOPROTECTIVE FOOD

Hepatoprotective foods are those foods that directly improve liver metabolism and health. For centuries, beets and fish (including fish oil) have been recognized for their liver-supportive benefits. There are several other foods with such properties, including:

- Beets.
- Spirulina.
- Fish oil, olive oil.
- Flaxseeds, chia seeds.
- Berries, especially blueberries, cranberries, and blackberries.
- Fruits, especially red grapes, grapefruit, cactus pear fruit.
- Garlic.
- Turmeric (Curcuma).
- Nuts, particularly walnuts.

These foods mostly fit into the *Green* or *Blue Baskets* (detailed in *Bonus 3*), and incorporating them into your diet early can shield your liver from toxins and inflammation while enhancing functions like bile production. Even so, removing toxic load is much more important than these "helpers."

 You cannot poison the organ and heal it at the same time.

Warning: A word of caution about Curcuma, also known as turmeric: While it's become quite a trendy supplement lately, taking too much over a long period, particularly in concentrated forms, may cause adverse side effects. However, sprinkling some turmeric spice into your meals, just as people have been doing for millennia across various cultures, is generally safe without the risk of overdose.

GLUTATHIONE

Maintaining your body's *glutathione* levels is key to keeping your liver's detox system running smoothly. Boosting your glutathione is as simple as choosing the right foods rich in this powerful antioxidant or encouraging your body to produce more of it. Here's a list of foods that can help:

- Sulfur-rich foods: cruciferous vegetables like broccoli, cauliflower, and cabbage, and allium vegetables, such as garlic and onions.
- Herbs and Spices: cilantro (also known as coriander), turmeric.
- Fruits: grapefruit, papaya, and pineapples.
- Peppers.
- Spinach.
- Avocados.
- Asparagus.
- Okra.
- Brazil nuts.
- Milk Thistle: Often taken as a supplement, be cautious with dosage.

Since glutathione is composed of three amino acids, a protein-rich diet is important to maintain adequate production in your body. Additionally, a healthy sleep routine is crucial, as lack of sleep can reduce glutathione levels.

Although some rare cases may benefit from glutathione supplements, consult your doctor to determine if they are appropriate for you.

See also:

• Key 5 ➤ Sleep and Circadian Rhythms

FOODS TO BOOST BILE PRODUCTION AND ENHANCE LIVER HEALTH

Certain foods boost your liver's overall health and function, or kick-start bile production directly. Spices are a great example—they can increase the production of stomach juices as well as bile. But here's the catch: this only works if your liver is healthy. You can ensure your liver's well-being by reducing toxic load and following the other steps we've discussed before.

Here's a list of powerhouse products you can add to your meals. Some directly stimulate bile production, others boost your liver's metabolism, and a few do both. You'll notice some familiar faces here —many of these are also great for improving stomach acidity. Basically, you're killing two flies with one swat.

- **N-3 Oils and Proteins:**
  - Olive oil.
  - Fatty fish (salmon, mackerel, sardines)
  - Nuts and seeds (almonds, walnuts, flaxseeds, chia seeds)
- **Vegetables:**
  - Beets
  - Cruciferous vegetables (broccoli, cauliflower, Brussels sprouts)
  - Leafy greens (spinach, kale, other dark leafy greens)
  - Celery
  - Garlic and onions
  - Artichoke
  - Jerusalem artichoke
  - Carrots
  - Radishes—any variety (including daikon, turnips)
- **Fruits:**

- Berries (especially blueberries, blackberries, cranberries, raspberries)
- Citrus fruits: Grapefruit, lemon, lime
- Apples
- **Herbs and spices:**
  - Turmeric, ginger, cinnamon, cumin, coriander, black pepper, fenugreek, sumac spice
  - Dill, cilantro, arugula, peppermint, fennel
- **Fermented vegetables and pickles.**
- **Herbal Teas:** hibiscus, chamomile
- **Supplements** (usually not necessary; consult with your doctor and be cautious about dosage):
  - Milk thistle
  - Dandelion root, Burdock root
  - Aloe vera
  - Ginseng

OTHER TACTICS FOR FIXING SIBO AND NORMALIZING MICROBIOME DISTRIBUTION

HEALTHY MOTILITY

Imagine a swiftly flowing mountain river, crystal clear and pristine. When its flow is unimpeded, it stays clean. Once it slows down or gets blocked, it begins to resemble a stagnant swamp, teeming with germs and parasites, with the previously clear water becoming unsafe to drink.

Similarly, in your digestive tract, passive intestinal motility mirrors the stagnant waters—a condition I call *Lazy Gut.* Just like a sluggish river encourages germs and parasites to thrive, a passive intestine does the same for pathogenic bacteria, giving them the perfect conditions to multiply and spread, often leading to *Small Intestinal Bacterial Overgrowth* (SIBO).

However, when your gastrointestinal tract's nerve and muscle cells work as they should, they create a dynamic flow, effectively controlling bacterial growth. This quick transit prevents bacteria from settling and multiplying excessively, thus avoiding overgrowth.

 Movement is Life.

Keep in mind that periodic *diarrhea* doesn't negate Lazy Gut; in fact, it's often a sign of it, tied to inflammation and poor absorption.

Reviving healthy gastrointestinal motility is a cornerstone of the 5R+ System, essential for immune system restoration. It is covered in depth in *Key 4*, where the tactics to help achieve this are discussed, but the primary factor for improvement is a healthy microbiome. Since gut movement and microbiome health are closely linked, tackling them together is essential to breaking out of the vicious cycle.

Addressing Lazy Gut is critical, and failing to do so can turn even beneficial prebiotics and probiotics into a problem. My advice is to exercise caution with these until you've made real progress on improving gut motility.

 Low Motility or Poor Digestion + Prebiotics = SIBO.

GUT FLUSHING EXERCISES FOR SIBO

Jumpstarting your SIBO recovery with specialized gut-flushing exercises offers quick relief by swiftly moving large amounts of harmful bacteria out of your system. See the step-by-step video guide in Key 4, and always perform this on an empty stomach.

Note: gut flushing doesn't pick and choose—it clears all types of bacteria. This is why it's especially useful for dealing with SIBO, where the small intestine's overgrowth is predominantly pathogenic. By flushing out these harmful bacteria and toxins, you reduce inflammation, free *ecosystem niches*, and clear the way for good bacteria to colonize. Think of gut flushing as weeding your garden. By removing the weeds, you've made space for other plants to grow. Leave that space empty too long, and the weeds come right back. Similarly, after a gut cleanse, it's vital to reintroduce beneficial *probiotics* promptly, filling up those newly available ecological niches and keeping the harmful bacteria at bay. For this, use a combination of *Probiotics*, herbs, and raw vegetables, including bitter ones.

While *gut flushing* is a strong start, it's not a standalone cure. The key lies in applying all the tactics mentioned earlier to cultivate a healthy *Microbiome Distribution*. For the best outcome, you might need multiple rounds of gut flushing followed by the reintroduction of probiotics and the consistent application of the 5R+ System.

See also:

• Key 4 ➢ Physical Activities for Optimal Bowel Transit ➢ Flushing the Gut: Ayurvedic Shankha Prakshalana Technique Simplified

• Key 1 ➢ Probiotics

• Bonus 2. The Art of Fermentation: Delicious Vegetable and Dairy Probiotics Recipes.

MEAL SPACING AND WATER-FASTING

Bacteria thrive on a constant supply of nutrients. Cut off their food supply, and growth stalls, while healthy motility moves them down the digestive tract. That's where a carefully planned fasting regimen can make a big difference.

A day or two of fasting with plenty of water, along with some moderate exercise to keep your digestive system active, can effectively combat *Small Intestinal Bacterial Overgrowth (SIBO)*. The trick here is to focus on hydration without eating, ensuring any bacterial overgrowth is flushed out rather than feeding on partially digested food.

Warning: If you have certain medical conditions, particularly diabetes, fasting requires careful monitoring and may not be for you—consult with your doctor first.

Spacing out your meals, a practice that echoes the principle of fasting, can also help. A highly effective, natural approach includes eating only early in the morning and around noon, then avoiding eating or snacking from midday until the following morning. Remember to drink plenty of water, starting at least 2-3 hours after your meal, to not interfere with digestion. This practice will keep the upper section of your digestive tract empty most of the time and discourage bacterial growth. This also supports intestinal epithelium health and facilitates motility. We'll explore this more in *Key 3*. This approach is essentially a form of *intermittent fasting*, a practice you might be familiar with. It's an age-old concept that's become quite popular again for its health benefits, which are numerous but beyond the scope of this book.

The beauty of adopting holistic, healthy lifestyle strategies lies in their comprehensive benefits—they enhance your overall health without unintended side effects. This sharply contrasts with medications, which may solve one problem but exacerbate others. That's why it's crucial to carefully manage drug dosages and closely observe your body's reactions to them, ensuring that the benefits outweigh the risks.

POWER OF HERBS, SPICES, AND OTHER FOODS TO CONTROL MICROBIAL Growth

One key factor of microbiome distribution problems, like SIBO, is a diet lacking components that slow down bacterial growth, instead offering a buffet of easy-to-digest nutrients for harmful bacteria. Nutrients shouldn't be a free-for-all—food should create something akin to an obstacle course to slow down microbial growth. This ensures bacteria multiply gradually as the food travels through your digestive tract.

> **Let your body's digestion, absorption, and motility functions dominate, not the germs.**

We've already explored how raw bitter vegetables play a crucial role in forming the microbiome's *Composition*. They're equally important for ensuring a balanced microbiome *Distribution*.

The essential oils, enzymes, and other bioactive components in many herbs and spices act as nature's antibacterial agents, regulating bacterial growth in the small intestine. Plants have evolved to produce these substances as a defense mechanism against bacterial and fungal invasions, ensuring they don't rot while still alive. The necessity for such defenses is particularly acute in warm, moist climates like India and Indonesia, which explains why many spices come from these areas. Yet, you'll find beneficial herbs and spices across the globe. When we eat these plants raw, we harness their antimicrobial power for our stomach and gut microbiome. Herbs and spices tackle bacteria in two ways: directly, through their chemical action on microorganisms, and indirectly, by improving digestion and promoting gut motility.

SPICES TO AVOID

Although spices enhance your microbiome's balance, be aware that certain spices might irritate or harm your stomach and gut lining. I suggest choosing spice varieties that don't cause such adverse reactions. Especially in your active healing phase, it's best to avoid these specific spices:

- Mustard.
- Horseradish and Wasabi.
- Hot peppers (including Chilli, Tabasco, Jalapeno, Serrano, and Cayenne).

If you decide to reintroduce them into your diet later on, do so slowly and use them in small amounts to avoid any adverse effects. Ideally, replace them with ginger, garlic, black pepper, and other spices.

ANTIMICROBIAL HERBS AND SPICES

Herbs offer many flavors and have the bonus of antimicrobial benefits, making them a great addition to any meal. Below are some of the most effective ones:

- Oregano
- Peppermint
- Spearmint

- Thyme
- Cilantro
- Dill
- Tarragon (estragon)
- Basil
- Rosemary
- Chive
- Marjoram
- Sage

In addition to these herbs, numerous spices also display remarkable antimicrobial properties. The following spices are generally safe and effective:

- Clove
- Cinnamon
- Garlic and onion
- Ginger (interestingly, studies show that ginger is especially effective when combined with artichoke.)
- Turmeric
- Coriander seeds
- Cumin
- Black pepper
- Bay leaves
- Cardamom
- Fennel seeds
- Berberis

While going for fresh herbs and spices is ideal, dried or frozen versions come in a close second, offering the benefits of a lengthy shelf-life and simple storage. It's easy to find these in bulk online, ensuring your pantry is always stocked. I find it very convenient to keep a collection of large jars with various dried herbs at hand to enhance my dishes.

> **Use herbs generously with all meals—it is not just about flavor but also changing the game with gut bacteria in your favor.**

Caution: *Artemisia* (Wormwood) and *Pau d'arco* (that's "bow tree" in Portuguese) are known for their potent antimicrobial and antiparasitic properties. However, these are not your typical culinary herbs; they're more like medicines and should only be used with proper guidance. I mention them only because you may encounter them in various health recommendations. Please consult your doctor if you decide to try them, as overdosing can pose significant risks.

N-Acetylcysteine (NAC)

You might have seen *N-acetylcysteine (NAC)* popping up in various health circles or promoted in ads. While it's not essential for our primary goals, this supplement can boost the antibacterial properties of many herbs and spices. NAC blocks the formation of *bacterial biofilms*—the tough shields bacteria build to fend off antimicrobial substances and enhance their chances of survival. By blocking the formation of biofilms, NAC strips bacteria of their protective barriers, rendering them more vulnerable to the power of antimicrobial agents.

Including NAC as a supplement can indeed enhance the power of herbs and spices right from the start of your regimen. It's optional, and you certainly don't need to use it long-term. Adding NAC can also tilt the balance in your favor in particularly stubborn SIBO cases that have shown little improvement over time.

As with any other supplement, I advise you to consult your health-care provider before starting NAC and carefully adhere to the recommended dosage.

DIE-OFF REACTIONS

Herxheimer reactions, often called *Die-off reactions*, are a common side effect when treating Small Intestinal Bacterial Overgrowth (SIBO). These reactions are your body's response to the release of toxins from countless dying SIBO bacteria. As these bacteria die off in large numbers, their released toxins are absorbed by your body, leading to a temporary state of intoxication. The worse the SIBO, the stronger the toxic reaction tends to be. These die-off reactions can last anywhere from a few hours to a week, heavily influenced by the rate of gut motility, which controls how quickly this toxic waste is expelled from your body. Your liver and kidneys are also involved in neutralizing and clearing these toxins from your bloodstream.

While experiencing these reactions can be uncomfortable, it indicates that the treatment is working and effectively reducing the harmful bacterial overgrowth.

SYMPTOMS OF DIE-OFF REACTIONS

The symptoms of a die-off reaction can vary significantly due to the variety of toxins released and the unique way each person's body reacts to them.

- General symptoms include:
  - Fatigue and a general sense of unwellness.
  - Brain fog or headaches.
  - Chills or fevers.
  - Muscle and joint pain.
  - Skin reactions like rashes or hives.
- Digestive symptoms might include:
  - Upset stomach.
  - Nausea or vomiting.
  - Gas or bloating.
  - Changes in stool frequency or consistency, including diarrhea or constipation.
  - Exacerbation of SIBO-related symptoms (like abdominal fullness, cramps, bloating, or constipation).

If you're experiencing these symptoms following a day or two of water fasting, you're likely dealing with SIBO, which must be addressed and treated promptly.

. . .

HOW TO TREAT DIE-OFF REACTIONS

One frequent recommendation is to combat SIBO gradually, aiming to avoid the flood of toxins that comes with rapid bacterial die-off. This strategy seeks to minimize severe reactions by prolonging bacteria elimination, which, while reducing the risk of acute intoxication, might extend your exposure to toxins, subtly causing more harm over time.

I advocate for a more straightforward method: if something's harmful, flush it out. Speeding up the removal of bacteria from your gut minimizes the absorption of toxins. Achieving this is easier with good gut motility (see *Key 4*). The aim is to remove dead bacteria swiftly.

Staying well-hydrated is critical to this approach. Drinking plenty of water promotes the active elimination of toxins. Another highly effective strategy involves a gut-flushing exercise circuit, as I explain in *Key 4*. This should only be done during water-fasting, to avoid sabotaging digestion and flushing down undigested food.

Using adsorbents like *activated charcoal* can also 'bind' the toxins, facilitating removal. Activated charcoal traps toxins, making them easier to eliminate, especially when followed by lots of water. You can take it as capsules or mix powder with water; doses typically range around 20-60 gram. Once you've taken the activated charcoal, give it 1-3 hours to work, then help cleanse your gut by drinking plenty of water and doing gut-flushing exercises. Reminder: check in with your healthcare provider first.

If toxins enter your bloodstream, your liver, kidneys, and sweat glands will work to eliminate them. Enhancing liver health, a topic we've touched on previously, is necessary to support this elimination process. Additionally, increasing sweating through sauna sessions can be an effective, natural way to expel toxins.

See also:

• Key 4 ➤ Flushing the Gut: Ayurvedic Shankha Prakshalana Technique Simplified

• Key 5 ➤ Hydrotherapy and Temperature Contrast

. . .

WHEN YOU MAY NEED LAXATIVE

Our primary approach leans heavily on tapping into the body's natural processes, steering clear of artificial interventions whenever possible. However, don't delay the removal of dead germs and toxins. If drinking plenty of water and doing gut-flushing exercises aren't enough to clear the die-off, consider other methods, like laxatives or enemas, to speed up the cleansing process.

While it's generally better to avoid them, over-the-counter *osmotic laxatives* might be justifiable for a one-off use under these exceptional conditions. Products such as *Milk of Magnesia, Polyethylene Glycol (PEG), Lactulose,* and *Magnesium sulfate (Epsom salt)* can be considered. If you have Crohn's disease or colitis, osmotic laxatives like *PEG* or *Lactulose* are often considered the best choice.

Warning: Consult your doctor before opting for these measures!

Frequent laxative use is not something I advocate. They can be helpful at the start of your healing, especially for dealing with die-off reactions from a major SIBO cleanup. After this initial phase, the goal shifts to preventing a return of these issues. By improving your gut motility, you likely won't need laxatives anymore. Once your gut motility is restored, your digestive system will keep up its good work, even if you go without food for a while.

See also:

• Key 4 ➤ Careful With Laxatives

INTEGRATED CLEAR-OUT STRATEGY

Once you've laid a solid foundation for your digestive system, tackling and wiping out SIBO becomes a more manageable task. Consider starting with oregano, mint, and other antimicrobial herbs, then follow up with a short fast lasting a couple of days. Support this regimen with plenty of water and gut-stimulating measures, choosing physical exercises over laxatives whenever possible. This quick-start method effectively flushes out bacterial overgrowth from your gut.

Maintaining active gut motility and optimal digestion afterward is critical to preventing SIBO's recurrence. Gradually reintroduce food with fiber-rich salads loaded with probiotics and prebiotics—raw leafy greens, bitter vegetables, herbs, spices, and naturally fermented foods, all lightly seasoned with olive oil and a splash of lemon or a drizzle of vinegar. Continue with this diet for a few weeks to fortify your gut health improvements. This strategy is most effective when your gut motility is already good, and adding more olive oil and *prokinetics* to your salads can help with that.

Typically, a focused and dynamic approach like this can significantly improve your gut microbiome *Distribution* and *Composition*.

See also:

• Key 4 ➤ Prokinetic and Laxative Foods

FUNGI: MOLD AND YEAST

SMALL INTESTINAL FUNGAL OVERGROWTH (SIFO)

Dealing with *Small Intestinal Bacterial Overgrowth* (SIBO) often means you're also up against its less talked-about companion, *Small Intestinal Fungal Overgrowth* (SIFO). In this condition, fungi, mainly mold and yeast, multiply excessively. These fungi cling to life stubbornly, making their elimination challenging. While treatment often takes longer, getting rid of them is definitely within reach.

Yeast, well-known for its role in brewing beer and baking bread, ferments carbohydrates by breaking them down into alcohol and carbon dioxide (CO_2). This fermentation is also a survival tactic: the alcohol produced can kill surrounding bacteria, giving yeast an advantage thanks to its remarkable alcohol tolerance. That's also why alcohol consumption negatively impacts *Microbiome Composition* in your gut. Molds play a similar game, releasing toxins that wipe out many types of bacteria, shrinking microbial diversity.

SIFO also impacts your liver and gut lining with powerful toxins.

FUNGAL SPORES: SOURCES AND TRANSMISSION

The primary triggers behind SIBO often also contribute to SIFO, with most cases being caused by low levels of gastric acid and bile, and passive motility. Moreover, antibiotics notoriously lead to fungal growth, whether they're medically prescribed or ingested indirectly through food.

Other culprits that might invite unwanted fungal spores into our gut include:

- **Alcohol** creates a *selective pressure* in the intestine, helping yeast outcompete beneficial bacteria. Moreover, alcoholic drinks, particularly **beer**, also contain yeast.
- **Moldy cheeses**—whether due to spoilage or as a feature in gourmet varieties.
- **Dried fruits** can be a hidden source of mold unless appropriately stored. If they look or smell strange, wash them thoroughly or discard them altogether.
- **Peanuts** are also prone to mold, especially when stored improperly or for too long. Roasting and shelling can reduce the risk, but always aim to keep nuts and peanuts in dry conditions.
- Your **living environment**—if the building has mold problems, spores can spread everywhere, affecting your health. It's crucial to address such issues promptly.

> Selective pressure is an environmental force that influences the survival and reproductive success of particular groups of organisms, favoring certain types while suppressing others. Over time, this pressure shifts the ecosystem's population, with some species thriving and others becoming extinct.

Stomach acid acts as a major barrier to fungal contamination. High stomach acidity levels can prevent mold from entering your gut, making your digestive system more resilient to external threats.

See also:
- Key 1 ➢ Probiotics
- Key 1 ➢ Stomach Acid
- Key 5 ➢ Microclimate: Small Changes Without a Big Move

. . .

BREAD — LEAVENED AND UNLEAVENED

Most bread varieties get their rise from yeast, a type of fungus. Although baking at high temperatures should, theoretically, kill all yeast, in practice, a small number of spores might survive due to uneven heat, the bread's shape, overly moist areas, or even post-baking contamination in the factory. That's why I typically suggest opting for flat, unleavened bread. They're not only yeast-free but also cook more thoroughly, reducing the chance of spore survival. You can find great examples all over the world, including Turkic lavash, Jewish matzo, Spanish tortillas, Indian and Pakistani roti or chapati, and French crepes.

Nevertheless, minimize your bread consumption. Whole-grain meals offer more nutritional benefits than bread.

See also:

• Key 1 ➤ Starch: From Protagonist to Bit Player

ADDRESSING THE SIFO PROBLEM

Tackling *Small Intestinal Fungal Overgrowth* (SIFO) often feels like navigating familiar yet more challenging terrain compared to *Small Intestinal Bacterial Overgrowth* (SIBO), which we discussed earlier. Even though managing SIFO involves strategies similar to the ones used with SIBO, it often demands more patience and effort to treat, requiring a longer and more intensive approach.

The key to managing SIFO is tweaking your diet. First, eliminate alcohol—it promotes yeast growth by enabling it to outcompete other microbes. Also, remove starch and sugar—yeast and mold feast on these carbs, turning your intestine into their preferred habitat. Especially during your active healing, you need to completely remove these foods from your diet to starve the fungi.

Switching to a diet abundant in greens and raw vegetables offers a healthy alternative. In severe cases of mold growth, saying goodbye to starchy foods isn't just advised—it's necessary. You might notice that this dietary shift echoes the popular "Paleo Diet" principles but with a twist: focus on plant-based choices.

Harness the power of bitter herbs and spices to tackle mold in the same way you do for SIBO.

Mold *die-off* resembles bacterial die-off but tends to hit harder. When managing it, the same strategies apply, with an increased emphasis on *gut flushing* to counteract the intense intoxication triggered by SIFO. In the most extreme cases, even medical intervention may be needed. Always consult with your doctor before choosing this path. However, I have observed that gut flushes can bring significant relief.

Last but not least, don't overlook the impact of fungal exposure in your living and working surroundings. *Key 5* has insights into this.

See also:

• Key 1 ➤ Feeding Your Enemies

• Key 1 ➤ Other Tactics for Fixing SIBO and Normalizing Microbiome Distribution

• Key 1 ➤ Die-off Reactions

• Key 4 ➤ Flushing the Gut: Ayurvedic Shankha Prakshalana Technique Simplified

• Key 5 ➤ Environment and Climate

FEEDING YOUR ENEMIES

Previous chapters covered how unhealthy digestion can disrupt our microbiome. In this chapter, we'll talk about other factors that can also negatively influence our internal ecosystem. One of the most common ways we inadvertently cause dysbiosis is by unintentionally fostering the growth of the microbes that should be scarce or absent. This happens when your diet consists mainly of nutrients that allow these microbes to flourish and outcompete the beneficial bacteria. The main culprit? Refined carbohydrates. A rare commodity in pre-industrial times, they unfortunately constitute a significant portion of modern diets.

 What you eat is not just nutrition for your body but also the environment for your microbiota.

SWEET DOES NOT EQUAL GOOD

SUGAR

Sugar is ubiquitous in today's food landscape. It sneaks into people's diets in various guises: from sucrose to fructose syrup, cane sugar to beet sugar, and organic sugar to brown sugar, infiltrating not just desserts but many other products, too.

We're all familiar with how sugar in the bloodstream affects our metabolism. Yet, in the digestive tract, the effects are less recognized, affecting your gut, microbiome, and immune health. When you indulge in a sugary cookie, your blood sugar level rises, so you go for a jog, thinking you'll burn off those extra calories. That's all very well and good, but the moment the sugar hits your gut, it begins reshaping your microbiota's environment. These changes persist long after your workout, regardless of how much you exercise or the size of your meal. Since sugar is their favorite food, pathogenic germs couldn't care less about your physical efforts. They flourish and multiply, shrinking the population of beneficial bacteria and creating health issues beyond weight gain.

Sure, opting for smaller cookies and more exercise will mitigate the metabolic harm, but the damage to your microbiome remains. This underscores the fact that the problem with sugar isn't just about extra pounds. The widespread belief that "low-sugar" is better because it contains fewer calories is a dangerous oversimplification.

That's why, if you have an active life, you should get your energy boost from healthy alternatives like complex carbohydrates, oils, and proteins, not sugar or refined starch.

The consumption of sugar has exploded over centuries. Once a rare luxury, its adverse health impacts were minimal due to its scant consumption by the wealthy few. Fast-forward from the 1700s to 2009, the average American's sugar intake has skyrocketed from 4.9 grams a day to an alarming 94 grams, with, by some estimates, almost half the population consuming up to 227 grams daily.

Sugar is now a common additive for flavor enhancement in many products, spurred by consumer preferences. Even as "low sugar" labels have become increasingly marketed, one has to wonder—low compared to what? Average? Yesterday's consumption? Our current "average" is already alarmingly high. The FDA's 50 grams per day sugar intake guideline seems more like a compromise between an ideal zero and our stark reality rather than a genuine health recommendation. Remember, these standards only consider the metabolic effects of food, ignoring the impact of sugar on our microbiome.

> **It is not"low sugar" you need, but zero added sugars.**

Because even the smallest amount of sugar can throw off the balance in your microbiome ecosystem, my advice is not to compromise. Look for healthy swaps for your sweet cravings later in this chapter. Don't be fooled by the marketing hype around brown organic sugar and the like as being healthier—brown sugar is still 96% sugar. Despite its higher mineral content, it's nutritionally similar to white sugar, making it just as harmful to your health. You should get your essential minerals from healthy whole food sources.

Does my advice to cut out sugar entirely sound too extreme? Consider this: is it not more extreme to eat your way onto the operating table? When viewed this way, it makes sense to choose olives over cookies for a treat.

NATURAL SWEETENERS

Since ancient times, people have been using natural sweeteners like honey, molasses (from dates, grapes, or carob), maple syrup, and agave syrup. However, the negative impacts of sugar on the microbiome we just discussed apply equally to these high-sugar alternatives.

> **Natural does not always mean healthy.**

In traditional cultures, this issue wasn't evident because the consumption of sweet foods was a rare event, limited to special occasions and feasts a few times a year. This limited exposure meant that the *selective pressure* exerted by sugars on the microbiome was minimal. The resilience of an otherwise healthy microbiome would prevail. That has changed. Today's access to and affordability of these natural sweeteners, coupled with a changed food culture, has led to much more frequent consumption.

Weekly, or even worse, daily indulging in even the most natural, highest quality, top-shelf triple-organic sweeteners can disrupt the microbiome, gut, and immune cells in much the same way as refined sugar. Even honey, often praised for its health benefits, has a couple of important considerations worth noting. Historically, honey was a rare and costly treat, and its occasional use allowed its nutritional and bioactive benefits to shine without the negative effects. Interestingly, wild honey from ancient times was significantly less sweet than the varieties we see now on supermarket shelves. The reason? Modern beekeeping practices—bee diets are often supplemented with sugar syrups to boost honey production, a perfectly legal, economically driven approach. As a beekeeper once shared with me: labels like "no sugar used" often mean fructose syrup was added instead, and if it mentions "no fructose syrup," then sugar or something similar was likely used. Without it, honey production would decrease significantly, turning beekeeping into a hobby rather than a commercial venture. Also, consider the potential risks from pesticide residues, which bees gather from treated plants, and the occasional use of antibiotics to treat bee diseases. In other words, today's honey is significantly different from its traditional, purely natural counterpart, making it the most affordable ever in history.

Switching from refined sugar to honey or natural syrups doesn't solve the issue of excessive consumption of sweet foods. It merely swaps one sugar source for another. It's our taste preferences and attitudes that need to change to halt the demand for added sugars in all kinds of foods.

ADDED SUGARS LABELS

Ever noticed that many food manufacturers often use sweeteners that, while not technically labeled as 'sugar'—a term reserved for table sugar or sucrose—are, in reality, just sugar in disguise? These can appear under many different names but have the same effect— they make food taste sweeter. Recognizing these ingredients enables you to make healthier food choices. Table 3.9 lists alternative names for added sugars you might encounter on labels.

Added Sugars Labels

- Agave nectar/syrup
- Barley malt
- Beet sugar
- Blackstrap molasses
- Brown rice syrup
- Brown sugar
- Buttered sugar
- Cane crystals
- Cane juice
- Cane sugar
- Caramel
- Carob syrup
- Castor sugar
- Coconut sugar
- Confectioner's sugar
- Corn sweetener
- Corn syrup
- Crystalline fructose
- Date sugar
- Demerara sugar
- Dextrin
- Dextrose
- Diastatic malt
- Ethyl maltol
- Florida crystals
- Fructose
- Fruit juice/nectars
- Galactose
- Glucose
- Golden sugar
- Golden syrup
- Grape sugar
- High-Fructose Corn Syrup (HFCS)
- Honey
- Icing sugar
- Invert sugar
- Lactose
- Malt syrup
- Maltodextrin
- Maltose
- Maple syrup
- Molasses
- Muscovado sugar
- Panela sugar
- Raw sugar
- Refiner's syrup
- Rice syrup
- Sorghum syrup
- Sucanat
- Sucrose
- Syrup
- Treacle
- Turbinado sugar
- Yellow sugar

Appendix 1: Table 3.9. Added sugars labels

UNNATURAL SWEETENERS

People's preference for sweetness strongly influences which products are available on grocery store shelves. With growing awareness about the health risks of added sugars, though, many are now seeking alternatives. This shift has led to a noticeable increase in the use of artificial sweeteners, chosen by those trying to reduce calorie intake or manage diabetes. These alternatives provide the sweetness people love without the added calories, making them a common ingredient in diet products. Yet, "no calories" doesn't mean "no problems." Most artificial sweeteners are not naturally processed by our bodies. Even though some "non-sugar" products are not synthetic, strictly speaking, they are still not a part of our healthy diet and metabolism, making them unnatural choices. Sweeteners and other food additives that are foreign to our microbiome and normal human biochemistry should not be a regular part of our food. A century ago, human organisms did not encounter them, so the potential risks are not yet fully understood, especially regarding their effects on gut bacteria. That's why these sweeteners are grouped with other *artificial food additives*, which I will cover in a future chapter.

The problem is that our food culture is stuck on the idea that "sweet equals tasty." When sugar's downsides became undeniable, we swapped it out for artificial substitutes, ignoring the fact that our bodies were not designed to handle these new chemicals. We've replaced one issue with another, overlooking the real solution: change the prevailing mindset that "sweet equals good."

 The culture that works against health ought to be changed.

Artificial sweeteners are now extensively used in processed foods, ranging from soft drinks and baked goods to candies, puddings, canned foods, jams, jellies, and even flavored dairy products.

The FDA has approved several nonnutritive sweeteners: *saccharin, aspartame, acesulfame potassium, sucralose,* and *neotame.* Yet, this green light only means no direct toxic effects have been detected. Such endorsement doesn't dismiss the possibility of unseen or delayed adverse effects, considering these additives are recent additions to human diets. Importantly, these evaluations do not measure the impact on our microbiome, which we know can indirectly affect the immune system and overall health.

See also:
• Key 1 ➤ Chemical Additives and Toxins in Our Food

Unnatural Sweeteners Labels

- Acesulfame Potassium:
  - ACK, Ace K, Equal Spoonful (also +aspartame), Sweet One, Sunett
- Aspartame:
  - APM, AminoSweet, Aspartyl-phenylalanine-1-methyl ester, Canderel (not in US), Equal Classic, NatraTaste Blue, NutraSweet
- Aspartame-Acesulfame Salt:
  - TwinSweet
- Cyclamate:
  - Calcium cyclamate, Cologran (cyclamate and saccharin), Sucaryl
- Erythritol:
  - Sugar alcohol, Zerose, ZSweet
- Glycerol:
  - Glycerin, Glycerine
- Glycyrrhizin:
  - Licorice
- Hydrogenated Starch Hydrolysate (HSH):
  - Sugar alcohol
- Isomalt:
  - Sugar alcohol, ClearCut Isomalt, Decomalt, DiabetiSweet (also contains Acesulfame-K), Hydrogenated Isomaltulose, Isomaltitol
- Lactitol:
  - Sugar alcohol

- Maltitol:
  - Sugar alcohol, Maltitol Syrup, Maltitol Powder, Hydrogenated High Maltose Content Glucose Syrup, Hydrogenated Maltose, Lesys, MaltiSweet (hard to find online to buy), SweetPearl
- Mannitol:
  - Sugar alcohol
- Neotame
- Polydextrose:
  - Sugar alcohol (Derived from glucose and sorbitol)
- Saccharin:
  - Acid saccharin, Equal Saccharin, Necta Sweet, Sodium Saccharin, Sweet N Low, Sweet Twin
- Sorbitol:
  - Sugar alcohol, D-glucitol, D-glucitol syrup
- Stevia:
  - Truvia, Pure Via, SweetLeaf, Splenda Naturals Stevia
- Sucralose:
  - 1',4',6'-Trichlorogalactosucrose, Trichlorosucrose, Equal Sucralose, NatraTaste Gold, Splenda
- Tagatose:
  - Naturlose
- Xylitol:
  - Sugar alcohol, Smart Sweet, Xylipure, Xylosweet

* Some of these ingredients are synthetic, while others, despite being plant-based, remain unnatural as regular components of the human diet.

Appendix 1: Table 3.10. Unnatural sweeteners labels

UNNATURAL SWEETENERS LABELS

I strongly suggest avoiding artificial sweeteners and other chemical food additives, often lurking behind a legion of commercial brand names. Make it a habit to always read the ingredients list before consuming any product.

See also:

• Appendix 1 ➤ Table 3.10

CONQUERING SUGAR CRAVINGS

You might think sugar cravings are just an inevitable aspect of life, but that's not the whole story. Sure, craving sweets is common, but it's not a natural or healthy reaction to hunger or food. It's actually a red flag, pointing to something off-balance that needs to be fixed.

A significant factor behind cravings for sweets is often an imbalance in gut bacteria. Yes, the state of your *microbiome* significantly affects your taste preferences. Another trigger is what's known as a *blood sugar crash*, caused by a hormonal imbalance resulting from... too much sugar. This sets off a rollercoaster of hormone and glucose level fluctuations, sparking a craving for even more sweets—a vicious cycle. Interestingly, the most subtle yet powerful driver of sugar cravings is *neuropsychological*, as these are deeply rooted in our brain's reward system, triggering responses similar to those seen in narcotic addiction. Yes, <u>sugar is addictive</u>.

Breaking free from sugar cravings requires more than willpower— it's about rebalancing your microbiota and diet. Following the 5R+ system can also significantly reduce these cravings by addressing the root causes directly. However, there's a psychological aspect too. Many of us have grown up associating sweets with rewards, celebrations, and comfort. To truly overcome sugar cravings, we must rethink and rewire these deep connections in our minds.

 The key is not just re-stocking the fridge but reshaping the mindset.

Developing a healthier taste and food culture takes deliberate action. Teach yourself that sweetness isn't a prerequisite for delicious-ness, and redefine your concept of dessert. Think outside the conven-tional dessert box and explore the rich flavors of different spices, herbs, and wholesome treats. Options like olives, nuts, pickles, or a piece of quality cheese, while not the usual dessert, can satisfy your sweet craving by fulfilling the psychological need for a yummy meal finale. Your goal is to break the association between sweetness and satis-faction.

 Be the master of your taste.

THE ABCS OF NATURAL SWEETS

Historically, the sweetest treats in our ancestors' diet were fruits—for millennia, nothing would replace the sweetness of dates, figs, or mangoes. Honey, as we've already seen, was an occasional luxury rather than a regular part of people's diets. This meant our sugar intake was naturally lower, and, more importantly:

 Normally, sweets come with a substantial dose of fiber.

When you eat sugars with fiber, it changes how they interact with your bacterial population. Fiber not only promotes healthy digestion and motility, but it also helps maintain a diverse gut microbiota and limits the growth of sugar-fed bacteria. Plus, fiber acts like a sponge and filter. Sweet fruits naturally offer a mix of sugar, fiber, and other nutrients, while many manufactured sweets, like pastries, lack fiber. Instead, they're packed with starch, which our digestive systems quickly convert into more sugar.

Eating sugar without balancing it with plenty of fiber is a hallmark of modern diets. It disrupts our gut microbiome composition and distribution and, research shows, can even directly trigger inflamma-tion. Understanding this enables you to make healthier dessert choices.

. . .

GOOD OPTIONS FOR SWEET CRAVINGS

Eliminating sweet snacks and desserts might seem daunting, particularly for individuals battling sugar addiction amidst a sea of tempting choices. Fortunately, there's a more straightforward approach that doesn't require the willpower of a Navy SEAL:

 Substitute instead of exclude.

Swap out sugary treats for wholesome, sweet alternatives, ensuring you're always well-stocked to satisfy any cravings. Top choices include fruits, nuts, and dried fruits. Slices of pineapple or papaya or a handful of berries, chestnuts, or pistachios can become your go-to dessert options.

From what I've observed, dried fruits can be particularly effective substitutes for sugary snacks due to their intense, concentrated flavor, pronounced sweetness, and the need for prolonged chewing. Despite their high sugar content, they also boast concentrated fiber and nutrients. This abundance of fiber changes how sugar interacts with your digestive system, benefiting your microbiome, gut health, and immune system.

The good news is that a huge variety of dried fruits is available online, far surpassing what you might find at your local grocery store. Virtually any fruit can be dried, giving you a vast arsenal to fend off cravings for unhealthy temptations. Plus, dried fruits are both shelf-stable and portable, making them a perfectly healthy option for travel or social gatherings. Keeping them on hand makes it possible for you to easily bypass the cake and ice cream—always carry a mix of dried fruits to swap the bad with the good.

 Love the food that loves you back.

Important: always ensure you buy *unsweetened* dried fruits, without added sugars. Some manufacturers add sugar to partially dried fruits as a preservative to make them softer and heavier—softer for taste and heavier to increase profit as they sell by weight. In this case, sweetened dried fruits aren't the healthy swap you want. Always check the label for added sugars or unnecessary additives.

See also:

- Key 4 ➤ The Fiber Paradox: Why Eat What You Can't Digest

CHILDREN'S FOODS — PASSING THE PROBLEM TO THE NEXT GENERATION

A child's relationship with food begins at an early age. Unfortunately, sugar often becomes a central part of that connection, sometimes with a nudge from well-meaning parents. Many commercially produced baby foods and children's meals are sweetened to boost their appeal to young taste buds. They are often marketed as "all-natural" because less refined sweeteners like juice concentrate, honey, or agave syrup are used. Despite the claim, these alternatives are much like sugar itself. Worse yet, these sweeteners can subtly steer children's taste preference towards added sweetness in everything they eat. Although born with a preference for sweetness—breast milk is sweet—infants don't naturally choose intensely sweet foods, nor do they gravitate to sweetness only. If encouraged to, they explore a variety of flavors, including bitter and sour vegetables and herbs. By guiding children to healthier options, we can help them develop a more balanced palate away from junk food.

 Sweet does not equal good.

Yet, many parents, supported by the food industry, unintentionally promote an unhealthy food culture in their children. They sweeten wholesome foods to disguise their natural flavors, using phrases like "it's sweet, so it's delicious" or "you won't even taste the [insert disliked food] because I added your favorite syrup." Thus, children grow up believing that doughnuts are better than olives and that ice cream is superior to chestnuts. They'll prefer sweetened yogurt over plain yogurt mixed with mint and minced garlic (an age-old treat and probiotic). These misconceptions influence their dietary choices into adulthood.

Furthermore, our society has deeply ingrained the idea that "sweetness is a reward," from ice cream parties to birthday cakes and candies as prizes for eating a salad. The message is clear and powerful—sweetness equals happiness. Children trust adults. This connection between treats and joy doesn't just fade away; it continues into adulthood. Supermarkets cleverly use this by tempting us with sweets at the checkout aisles.

This cultural norm, combined with sugar's addictive neurophysiological effects, disrupts people's gut microbiota, contributing to allergies and compromising their immune systems. Shockingly, various estimates show that between 25% to 40% of US children suffer from some form of allergies, with long-term consequences including higher risks of autoimmune diseases and cancer. Furthermore, sugary foods have been associated with metabolic disorders, cardiovascular diseases, and cognitive impairment.

 Physiologically, your body hates sugar, regardless of your taste preferences.

It also dampens the appreciation for healthier foods. Ever notice how kids often bypass vegetables, particularly the bitter ones, essential for maintaining a healthy microbiome and digestion? They may even prefer artificial sweets to natural fruits due to the more intense flavor of the former. This trend has shifted the fruit market towards sweeter varieties, leading to the decline, for example, of sour or tangy apples and berries and reducing valuable bitter phytonutrients in modern grapefruit cultures. Almost all modern vegetables have been bred to be sweeter and less bitter than their ancient varieties, which means they are lower in *polyphenols* and higher in carbohydrates. As plant breeders cater to consumer taste preferences, the diversity and nutritional benefits nature offers us are dwindling.

Yes, we cannot make the producers and sellers of sweetened foods for children pay their customer's future medical bills. However, we can steer little ones towards healthier eating habits while they cannot make educated choices themselves.

STARCH: FROM PROTAGONIST TO BIT PLAYER

Starch, a prevalent carbohydrate in our diet, quickly turns into sugars in the digestive system. It also promotes the growth of non-beneficial bacteria. Too much starch can throw your microbiome off balance. But here's an exciting twist: not all starches are created equal. *Resistant starch* breaks down more slowly and primarily feeds bacteria in the lower parts of the intestine, improving your colon microbiome and overall digestive health.

When consumed in moderation, starch is a generally beneficial nutrient and source of energy. However, don't let it take center stage in your meals. Striking the right balance means consuming just enough to fuel your body without creating a welcoming environment for pathogenic bacteria, yeast, and mold that feast on starch. This is where the 5R+ framework becomes invaluable, helping to shift the balance towards a healthier you. But remember, even if your microbiome, gut epithelium, and motility are in top shape, excessive starch intake can still tip the scales in the wrong direction.

To better illustrate this, I've categorized starchy foods into four groups based on their starch content and nutritional value—See Table 3.11.

Modern bread has come a long way from the traditional bread of the days of yore. It's often made from refined, sometimes bleached flour and frequently contains additives for extended softness and shelf life. While traditional whole-grain bread belonged to **Group 2b**, today's refined-flour bread falls into **Group 3**.

My advice is straightforward: eliminate **Group 3**, the unnatural, refined starches. For example, replace bread with options like oats or cooked whole grains. However, some grains may not be tolerated until your intestinal lining is well-repaired. In particular, you may need to avoid those containing *gluten*. Better yet, fill your plate with **Group 1** foods and limit those from **Group 2**. I've seen significant improvements in autoimmune conditions when people entirely cut out **Group 2** foods, focusing instead on **Group 1** and, even more so, on greens, bitter vegetables, and herbs during the active healing phase.

Starchy Foods

Nutritious natural foods—rich in starch, including resistant starch, and packed with protein, fiber, and other essential nutrients.	1. Most nutritious	• Pulses
		  ◦ Lentils
		  ◦ Beans
		  ◦ Peas
		  ◦ Chickpeas
		• Chia
		• Quinoa

Natural foods high in starch but with lower levels of resistant starch and less protein and other nutrients.	2a. More nutritious	• Grains:
		  ◦ Wheat
		  ◦ Rice
		  ◦ Oats
		  ◦ Buckwheat

	2b. Less nutritious	• Corn
		• Starchy tubers:
		  ◦ Potatoes
		  ◦ Sweet potatoes
		  ◦ Yams

Processed starchy foods made from refined carbohydrates that lack resistant starch and other beneficial nutrients.	3. Not nutritious	• Bread • Various bakery products • Pasta • Crackers • Refined flours

Appendix 1: Table 3.11. Starchy foods categories

As you start feeling better, it's safe to cautiously reintroduce some **Group 2** foods, especially those from **Group 2a**. Remember, they're not the stars of your diet—they're there just to complement it. Approach **Group 2b** with even more caution due to its low nutrient density. The truth is, you will not miss out on any essential nutrients or food variety by completely eliminating **Group 2b** and, especially, **Group 3** from your diet. Ideally, you want to balance starch in your diet with lots of fiber, much like you do with natural sugar consumption. This becomes especially crucial for low-fiber starchy foods beyond **Group 1.**

If you're tackling *Small Intestinal Fungal Overgrowth* (SIFO), cutting out starchy foods is non-negotiable during the entire healing stage. That's because starch is the primary substrate for fungal and mold growth. Instead, focus your diet on greens, herbs, and those all-important bitter vegetables.

Have you noticed that the typical Western diet flips these healthy principles, favoring refined carbohydrates instead of whole grains? You'll find that **Group 3** and **Group 2b** foods often dominate the plates, making up to half of the daily intake. While this may be cheap, it's a raw deal for your health.

 Ideally, more than half of your diet should be raw vegetables, fruits, nuts, and seeds.

See also:
- Appendix 1 ➤ Tables 3.11, 5.3
- Key 3 ➤ Eliminate Obstacles ➤ Obstacle #4: Harmful Food Ingredients ➤ Gluten

OTHER RISKS TO YOUR MICROBIOME HEALTH

The *Distribution* and *Composition* of your microbiome are closely intertwined. Healthy digestion aids Distribution by mitigating conditions like Small Intestinal Bacterial Overgrowth (SIBO). This, in turn, supports the beneficial bacteria in your gut and inhibits the harmful ones, enhancing your microbiome's Composition. Having a rich, diverse microbiota enhances your gut's functions, from improving motility to boosting digestive enzymes production, all crucial for optimal Distribution. It's like two sides of an arch supporting each other—if one side falters, the whole structure is at risk. SIBO, for example, deprives beneficial bacteria downstream of necessary nutrients and suppresses them with toxins, leading to a less diverse microbiota. Any disturbances in Distribution can negatively impact Composition, and vice versa. This explains the importance of simultaneously applying all 5R+ strategies to avoid deadlocks.

As we've seen earlier, added sugars and too much starch can wreak havoc on the microbiome, affecting both its Distribution and Composition. But it doesn't stop there—several other factors can also lead to Composition issues, either by quickly killing off good bacteria or slowly promoting harmful ones through *selective pressure*.

These factors include:

- Intestinal inflammation.

- Oral microbiota issues.
- Antibiotics.
- Chlorine, chloramine, and other disinfectant residues in water.
- Harmful food ingredients and toxins.

INFLAMMATION

Hidden, chronic inflammation in the intestine often helps aggressive bacteria dominate. As these harmful microbes multiply, they cause further damage to the epithelial cells, leading to increased inflammation. Adopting an anti-inflammatory diet contributes to a healthier environment for the gut microbiome, thereby breaking this vicious cycle. This book's *Key 2* section offers more insights on this important topic.

ORAL MICROBIOTA

Your *oral microbiota* is important for overall health, second only to the *gut microbiome*. These two microbial communities, each found in different parts of the same system, constantly interact with and influence each other. In *Key 5*, I will cover what you can do to improve the state of the microbiome in your mouth.

See also:
- Key 5 ➤ Oral Health and Other Autoimmune Triggers

ANTIBIOTICS

Antibiotics act like bombs on the microbiome, decimating beneficial bacteria and leaving empty spaces for opportunistic pathogens to take over. This can quickly and dramatically disrupt the microbiome.

Not long ago, I observed a similar scenario in my backyard. A landscaping project stripped away the top layer of grass and soil to improve water drainage, exposing the bare ground beneath. Within a few days, weeds started staking their claim on what used to be my well-maintained lawn. The solution was rapid action: covering the bare patches with new grass sods to rehabilitate the area.

It's important to note that antibiotics don't eliminate every germ. They tend to leave behind the most aggressive and resistant ones, giving them an edge to dominate, often at the expense of the beneficial bacteria that might not be as resistant and are easily destroyed. As a result, antibiotics can significantly reduce the diversity of your micro-biome. Even small exposures to antibiotics over time create a *selective pressure* that shifts the composition of the microbial population, explaining the prevalence of tough-to-treat 'superbugs' in hospital settings.

Physicians are increasingly cautious with antibiotic prescriptions, recognizing their impact on the microbiome. After necessary antibiotic treatment, it's vital to support the microbiome's recovery with probi-otics and to counter potential fungal infections (like yeast and mold) with antifungals. Fungi, which are resistant to antibiotics, are normally controlled by a strong and diverse microbiota. However, when antibi-otics disrupt this balance or if the immune system is weakened, the risk of fungal infections increases.

Always talk to your healthcare provider about potential alterna-tives to antibiotics. However, if you need to take them, it's crucial to follow a plan to rebuild your healthy microbiome quickly.

ANTIBIOTICS RESIDUES IN FOOD

It's a known fact that antibiotics can sneak into our bodies through the food we eat. Livestock are often given antibiotics to fight infections and promote growth. This might sound odd, but the change antibiotics trigger in animals' microbiomes can cause them to gain weight—bad for their health but good for the farming industry. Indeed, human obesity is similarly linked to changes in the microbiome, suggesting that the 5R+ System can help with weight loss. Many people experi-ence this paradox—eating small portions and spending hours on the treadmill, unable to shed the stubborn extra pounds. For them, reshaping the microbiota can be the missing link.

In 1989, the Institute of Medicine estimated that about half of the

31.9 million pounds of antimicrobials consumed in the U.S. weren't for treating sick people or animals but for boosting growth in livestock. Fast forward to 2022, and that figure has jumped: nearly 70% of all medically essential antibiotics in the U.S. are now earmarked for agriculture.

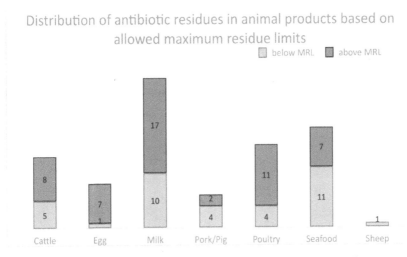

Distribution of antibiotic residues in animal products based on allowed maximum residue limits

Appendix 1: Figure 3.12 - Antibiotic residues in animal products based on allowed maximum residue limits (MRL). Source: https://www.mdpi.com/2079-6382/10/5/534

In the U.S., regulations cap how much antibiotic residue can be left in animal products. Still, sometimes, products end up with more than what's allowed. While these slip-ups don't happen often, the real worry is the effects of even tiny amounts of antibiotics on the human microbiome when consistently ingested over a long time. Current legal standards on how much antibiotic residue is okay don't consider what this might do to our microbiome. This gap in the regulations is partly because we're still learning about the microbiome and partly because keeping things this way is very profitable for large corporations.

See also:

• Appendix 1 ➢ Figures 3.12, 3.13

EFFECT OF ANTIBIOTICS ON MICROBES IN ANIMAL PRODUCTS

Beyond the residual antibiotics lingering in our food, there's another, often overlooked, issue that directly impacts us: the negative changes to the animals' microbiomes, which we unknowingly inherit through our diet. The widespread use of antibiotics in modern industrialized farming—to boost growth, prevent disease, and treat infections— significantly impacts the animals' microbiota. Livestock raised under these conditions aren't as robust as those in the wild or raised traditionally, leading to compromised health. These issues are then transferred to us via germs in dairy, meat, and eggs. Even though the contamination may seem minimal, and very few of these resistant bacteria make it through, their gradual accumulation over time poses a real threat to our well-being.

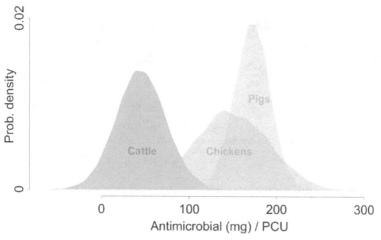

Appendix 1: Figure 3.13 - Estimates of antimicrobial consumption in cattle, chickens, and pigs in OECD countries. Source: https://doi.org/10.1073/pnas.1503141112

When livestock are given antibiotics, it leads to *antibiotic-resistant bacteria* in food products, which can disrupt our healthy microbiome. Research shows how disturbing this trend is. A 2001 study that examined 200 samples from U.S. grocery stores found that 20% of chicken, beef, turkey, and pork had Salmonella, and 84% of those were resistant to at least one antibiotic. A decade later, a similar study found that 81% of ground turkey, 69% of pork chops, 55% of ground beef, and 39% of chicken breasts, wings, and thighs sold in U.S. supermarkets carried antibiotic-resistant bacteria. In another 2011 study, scientists examined 136 samples of beef, poultry, and pork from 36 supermarkets across the U.S. Astonishingly, nearly a quarter of these samples contained antibiotic-resistant bacteria. These "superbugs," originating from modern industrial farms, can become your gut's *invasive species*, disrupting the natural microbiota.

Navigating Animal Products

If you're vegan, the issue of antibiotics in animal microbiomes won't affect you. However, for meat eaters and dairy lovers, it's vital to make informed choices. Seek out products labeled as raised without hormones and antibiotics, especially for dairy, which is often eaten raw. Also, cook your meats and eggs thoroughly to eliminate any remaining bacteria. Slightly undercooking your meat might not seem like a big deal, but over time, the effects of residual bacteria accumulate. This concern escalates when the bacteria are from animals treated with antibiotics, as they tend to be more resistant and aggressive strains you'd rather not have in your gut.

Recall our discussion on *Conquest vs Immigration*. Food safety standards aim to prevent severe bacterial outbreaks that can lead to immediate health problems (the *Conquest* scenario), not necessarily the subtle, long-term changes to your microbiome from minor bacterial exposures (*Immigration*) or *selective pressure*.

The amount of antibiotics used varies by animal type. Estimates suggest that pigs and poultry top the list, with 172 mg and 148 mg of antimicrobials used per kilogram of animal produced, respectively. Cattle are lower on the scale at 45 mg, while goats and sheep receive substantially fewer antibiotics, potentially making their meat and dairy a safer choice. This highlights that cheaper options are not always the best for your health.

 Prioritize quality over quantity, particularly when it comes to animal products.

Finding animal products from livestock that haven't been treated with antibiotics or hormones (we'll touch on the latter soon) can be quite a task. If you can not find such items, consider cutting them out entirely, especially during the active healing phase. Evidence suggests that eggs, dairy, and meat often have an inflammatory effect, giving you another reason to step back from them. But don't worry—there's a world of plant-based proteins and fish options to explore, so you won't miss out on protein. Once your gut microbiota is restored, you can be more flexible with your diet. A diverse, robust microbiome can handle the occasional dietary indulgence. But as a rule of thumb:

 Choose animal products from healthy animals that have never been given unnatural additives.

See also:
• Key 1 ➢ Overcoming Microbiota Inertia: Conquest or Immigration
• Appendix 1 ➢ Figures 3.12, 3.13

CHLORINE AND RELATED COMPOUNDS IN WATER

Now, let's talk about something that often flies under the radar but can significantly impact your gut microbiota—the residuals in municipal water. The tap water we drink and cook with goes through extensive treatment, often including *chlorine* and similar agents, to kill off water-borne infections and ensure it's safe to drink. Although chlorine disinfectants are largely eliminated during water treatment, trace amounts can still be found in our tap water. As with many other things, officially, the levels left are considered safe, but here's the catch: those safety measures only consider what's necessary to avoid acute or chronic poisoning in humans, not the *selective pressure* of the chemicals on the microbiome. The long-term, low-level exposure to these residuals can gradually erode the diversity of your gut microbiome and suppress the growth of beneficial bacteria.

I will return to the role of hydration in later chapters—water is irreplaceable, and drinking plenty of it is non-negotiable for your health.

That's why filtering your water, both for drinking and cooking, is essential to eliminate even the tiniest traces of chemical contaminants.

Chlorine is commonly used for water treatment, but many companies now use *chloramine*, which lasts longer than chlorine and provides a more stable defense against germs. While chloramine may be more effective for preventing infections, removing it from water is more challenging.

Your strategy for ensuring clean water at home will depend primarily on whether your local water supply uses chlorine or chloramine. Standard high-quality water filters can handle chlorine well, but dealing with chloramine requires a more specialized solution. It's best to check with your municipality to understand what's in your water.

Standard filters, like those in pitchers, under-sink systems, or fridge doors, mainly use activated carbon. This type works well for removing chlorine, but for chloramine, you'll need filters that use catalytic carbon. So, if your local water treatment includes chloramine, you'll need a more advanced system specifically designed to tackle this chemical. Check the technical specifications and laboratory results of any filter you consider—don't rely solely on marketing claims.

If you live somewhere where boiling your water before use is the norm, a quick boil can eliminate chlorine because it evaporates easily. If you use a wide pot, it'll go faster, thanks to a greater surface area. But if your water contains chloramine, boiling it away isn't so simple. You'd need to keep it bubbling for over 20 minutes, something nobody does.

When it comes to bottled water, it's not just the purification process that matters. Many brands use ozone treatment, which is both safe and effective. The genuine concern often lies with the bottle itself. Be especially wary of bottles made from materials that can leach *bisphenol-A (BPA)* into the water. Moreover, all plastic bottles have the risk of shedding *microplastics* into the water, a topic we explore later. Glass-bottled water doesn't have such problems.

See also:

• Key 1 ➤ Chemical Additives and Toxins in Our Food

• • •

REVERSE OSMOSIS AND REMINERALIZATION

Reverse osmosis (RO) filtration systems are top-notch for purifying water and removing almost everything, from chlorine and chloramine to heavy metals and microplastics. In recent years, they have gained popularity for home use thanks to increased affordability and simplicity. But there's a catch: they also remove vital minerals, resulting in nearly pure H_2O—something quite different from the natural water our bodies are used to. Drinking water that's been completely demineralized can be harmful in the long run, potentially affecting your intestinal mucous membrane and even contributing to cardiovascular disorders.

You might think, "Well, I can get those minerals from food or supplements," and you're right. But that's not the whole story. The real issue with demineralized water, which lacks salts and minerals, is that it is *hypoosmotic*. This means it has fewer *electrolyte* particles compared to the fluids inside your body cells, potentially leading to *hypotonic stress*. A big difference between the electrolyte concentration outside versus inside the cells can cause damage to the cell membranes. More water seeps into the cells, causing them to swell and damaging their internal structure. That's why drinking distilled water isn't recommended. While occasional consumption will do no harm, the long-term effects of drinking demineralized water can impact the health of your gut epithelium—a crucial component of the DILL+ framework that we must repair (as outlined in *Key 3*).

Naturally, we should drink mineral water. So, what's the solution? If using a reverse osmosis system, add some minerals back to your water. You don't need to include every single mineral (*microelement*)—a balanced diet and some food supplements should cover that. What's important is reintroducing essential electrolytes like calcium, magnesium, potassium, or sodium to counteract the water's *hypotonicity*, making it very slightly salty, as spring or mineral water would be. This will protect your gut epithelium cells from potential damage.

You have several options to remineralize your water effectively:

- Use a filter with a remineralization stage. This add-on cartridge reintroduces essential minerals into the water after it's been purified by reverse osmosis. Many filtration systems allow for the inclusion of a remineralization step without a complete system overhaul.

- Consider an "alkaline pitcher." They provide an easy way to add minerals back into water that's been distilled or treated by reverse osmosis. Make sure the one you choose is genuinely designed for remineralization, not just taste enhancement.
- Concentrated mineral drops are another practical solution. Just a few drops can transform a jar of filtered water into mineral water. It's an affordable option, but choosing a reputable brand is vital as the market is flooded with low-quality, dubious products.

Whichever remineralization method you choose, check the source of the mineral salts to avoid contamination with arsenic or other heavy metals. Independent lab tests can provide assurance, so prioritize products backed by transparent and reliable analyses and beware of deceptive marketing claims.

WHY WATER QUALITY MATTERS

It might seem like I'm making a big deal out of nothing—it's just water, after all. Why worry about tiny residues you can't see, taste, or smell? The point is we consume more water than anything else. It's important for hydration and maintaining health. Over the years, even tiny amounts of these residues add up to have cumulative effects on your well-being.

 Given our daily high water consumption, its quality is paramount.

Research highlights a link between the quality of local mineral water sources and longer life spans across different regions. Also, water that's too soft or has imbalanced fluoride concentrations can harm dental health, and traces of arsenic can cause manifold diseases, including cancer. So, it is no surprise that the 'safe' levels of disinfectants like chlorine or chloramine may still disrupt your gut microbiome and, by extension, your immune system.

Every year, I research the latest market offerings for water filtration and remineralization solutions and compile the findings to share with my subscribers. To access this annual report, join our community at www.autoimmunityunlocked.org .

CHEMICAL ADDITIVES AND TOXINS IN OUR FOOD

Two kinds of substances in your food, even if consumed in tiny amounts, can significantly impact your microbiome:

- **Food additives**: substances deliberately added to food to improve its taste, aroma, appearance, and overall sensory appeal.
- **Toxins**: substances not intentionally added to food; they often enter our food through environmental chemical pollution or industrial processes.

Food additives and unintentional toxins share a common trait—they're often foreign to the body's processes. Unlike essential nutrients like vitamins or polyphenols, they are not needed for our biochemical functions. Your body looks at these unfamiliar molecules with bewilderment, like a meticulous housekeeper confronting mysterious, unidentifiable objects. Even if not directly poisonous, they are perceived as clutter—chemical garbage serving no purpose. Some food additives, created synthetically, were nonexistent in human diets just a century ago and were introduced into food production mainly to boost industry profits. Business and culinary motives aside, to your body—they are all harmful.

The liver, your primary defense against toxins entering the bloodstream, is affected by all these substances, impacting functions like bile production. These ingredients also usually harm the digestive tract epithelium. Their safety levels are regulated by policies that stipulate "permissible limit concentrations," based on their direct impact on human health. However, these recommended restrictions completely disregard the chemicals' effects on our gut microbiome—a field that has only recently gained attention.

Even tiny concentrations of *food additives* and *toxins* can create *selective pressure* on your gut microbiota, encouraging some bacteria growth while inhibiting others, leading to a less diverse microbiome. The extent to which they disrupt the microbiome and impact our immune health is still largely unknown and not fully understood.

 The established safety levels for food additives and toxins do not consider the selective pressure exerted on the microbiome.

CHEMICAL TOXINS IN A POLLUTED WORLD

Due to increasing industrial pollution, chemical toxins in our environment—and thus our food supply—have become a pressing concern. A 2021 United Nations report unveils a frightening reality: over one-third of the world's farmland is chemically contaminated. This makes it more critical than ever to pay attention to your food's origin, including how and where animals are raised and fed and where your fish is sourced.

In today's globalized world, your food can come from almost anywhere, and standards for environmental cleanliness vary significantly from one country to the next. Some have been more effective at reducing chemical pollution, enforcing strict regulations, and offering relatively safer food sources. Navigating the complex landscape of food safety demands both diligence and knowledge. It's about learning which countries and regions maintain lower levels of chemical pollution and higher levels of food safety control.

While completely dodging chemical toxins might seem like a Herculean task, there are a few practical steps you can take to minimize your exposure.

Sidenote: While many contaminants have a more direct impact on the liver, gut lining, and other organs than on the microbiome, their effects significantly influence all DILL+ factors, including the microbiome and the immune system. That's why we'll explore these topics further in this chapter.

ORGANIC PRODUCE

Choosing organic food is a smart strategy. While standards vary internationally, organic certification typically means the product was:

- Grown without synthetic fertilizers, pesticides, herbicides, or chemicals.
- Cultivated in soil free from synthetic chemicals.
- Processed and stored without synthetic chemicals.

However, remember that "organic" doesn't necessarily guarantee better taste, appearance, or nutrient content.

Prioritize choosing organic options for foods most frequently contaminated with chemicals, such as:

- Meat and poultry
- Dairy products
- Leafy greens and other green vegetables
- Root vegetables
- Green beans
- Peppers
- Berries

Opting for organic versions of these foods can significantly reduce your exposure to harmful chemical contaminants.

MICROPLASTICS AND NANOPLASTICS

Let's discuss something that's been quietly affecting our food and, ultimately, our health for the past 100 years: *microplastics*. While these toxins primarily target the liver and other organs instead of the micro-biome, their relevance to food safety makes them worth mentioning here.

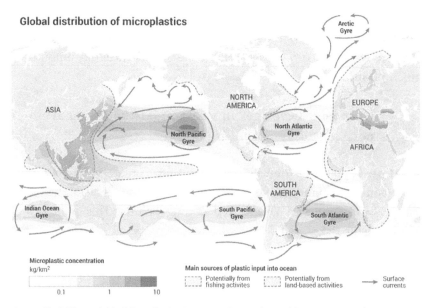

Appendix 1: Figure 3.14 - Microplastics in oceans. Source: https://www.grida.no/resources/13339

Since 1907, humanity has produced over nine billion tons of plastic —almost all of it is still with us. That's because plastic isn't like the leaves in your backyard that are biodegradable and decompose; it just breaks down into smaller and smaller pieces. These bits, called *microplastics* and *nanoplastics*, can be tinier than a grain of sand or even a cell. They are now found in every corner of the globe, including our oceans and seas. Check out the maps in Appendix 1. Alarmingly, plastic particles are also being detected in every human organ and tissue.

Our plastics problem comes full circle when animals eat these tiny pieces, and plants absorb nanoplastics from the soil. Nature eventually brings our plastic rubbish back to us in the form of microscopic parti-cles hidden in our food. While plants are generally the safest, fish and seafood often carry the highest levels of contamination, something we'll cover shortly. So, if you are vegan, you already minimize this risk.

Unfortunately, it doesn't stop there: our bottled water isn't safe either. Those plastic bottles? They can release microplastics and nanoplastics into the water they hold, especially if stored for a long time or exposed to sunlight. So, what can you do? Try to avoid bottled water or run it through a filter to reduce the amount of microplastics.

 Keep your beverages in steel or glass bottles to avoid microplastics.

Hint: Replace all utensils that come into contact with your food with non-toxic materials, such as glass food containers, stainless steel bottles, and wooden spatulas and cutting boards. This will further minimize the risks.

See also:
• Appendix 1 ➤ Figure 3.14

FISH SAFETY

Most human-produced waste, especially plastic, ends up in the ocean, breaking down into tiny fragments that sea creatures eat. While this pollution is a pervasive global issue, its severity varies by location. That's precisely why you need to know the origins of your fish and whether it's wild-caught or farm-raised.

Let's take a closer look at the areas most affected by pollution:

• The *Great Pacific Garbage Patch*, a massive floating waste site in the North Pacific Ocean, contains up to six times more plastic than marine life, covering an area double the size of Texas.
• Similar plastic and chemical pollution zones also plague the Indian Ocean and North Atlantic.
• The Mediterranean and Caribbean seas are also heavily impacted by pollution.

- The seas surrounding China and India, including their rivers, are significantly polluted by industrial waste and dense populations.
- Generally, water bodies near urban or industrial areas carry high pollution levels. For this reason, most freshwater fish in the contiguous United States are unsafe for consumption.

On the brighter side, some areas are in far better shape:

- The Arctic and Antarctic regions
- Certain areas of the South Pacific and South Atlantic oceans

Fish caught in these waters are less likely to be contaminated.

The safety of farmed fish depends on how they're raised and where. Different countries have different safety standards. For instance:

- Norway, Iceland, Australia, Scotland, and New Zealand adhere to higher farming standards.
- Lower standards are common in fish farms in China, India, Thailand, Vietnam, and Indonesia.

To clarify: wild-caught fish is not always better than farmed. Also, consider geography and environmental management. Fish from a farm with good quality control and sound farming practices in an ecologically clean area is much better than wild catch from the South China Sea or Mississippi River, for example, which are heavily polluted with industrial waste.

The type of fish also matters when it comes to contamination. Larger predatory species like sharks, halibut, catfish, and tuna tend to gather more pollutants due to their longer life spans. Smaller fish usually have less contamination. Shellfish, however, also tend to carry higher levels of toxins.

HEAVY METALS AND CHELATION FOODS

Lead, mercury, arsenic, and cadmium are the heavy metals most commonly associated with health issues. Ingesting them through food or water can cause a range of problems, from autoimmune diseases to liver and kidney damage and even cancer.

To safeguard against this, start with your tap water. Have it tested, and if you find heavy metals or other contaminants, invest in a high-quality water filter. The need to filter out chlorine compounds was highlighted earlier, and the same principles apply to heavy metals.

Remember that fish can also accumulate heavy metals throughout their lives. Large predatory fish and those from industrially polluted areas pose the highest risks. To navigate these waters safely, follow the advice given above on *Microplastics* and *Fish Safety*.

In the plant kingdom, rice has a knack for absorbing both the good and the not-so-good stuff from the soil. While it can be a great source of minerals like zinc and magnesium, rice grown in contaminated soil can also pick up high levels of heavy metals. Brown rice, being less processed, tends to contain more minerals, which unfortunately includes heavy metals if the soil is contaminated.

The risk of heavy metal contamination isn't the same everywhere. In the southeast U.S., arsenic-based pesticides were once common in cotton fields. Nowadays, rice grown in these areas may absorb that leftover arsenic. Yet, rice from the western U.S. and many regions of Pakistan and India typically has lower arsenic levels and is a safer alternative. Check out the maps in *Appendix 1* for a general overview of soil contamination by heavy metals across the U.S.

There are also a few easy kitchen tricks that can help reduce the heavy metal content in your rice:

- Always rinse your rice thoroughly before cooking, and consider pre-soaking it.
- Cook it in plenty of water.
- Drain off the excess water after cooking.

Eliminating heavy metals from the body isn't easy. However, certain foods with *chelating properties* can naturally boost your body's ability to expel these contaminants:

- Chlorella.
- Kelp.
- Blueberries.
- Cilantro.
- Garlic and other alliums.
- Fiber-rich vegetables and greens.

Even though these natural chelators can help purge heavy metals, it's essential to seek medical advice if you believe you've been significantly exposed. Sometimes, professional treatments like *chelation therapy* might be necessary.

See also:

- Appendix 1 ➤ Figures 3.15, 3.16, 3.17

ALCOHOL

Alcohol, despite its cultural popularity, is essentially a toxin. Our liver works hard to process and neutralize it, even when consuming small amounts. Beyond the well-known effects on the liver, alcohol severely impacts gut health. It also drastically diminishes the diversity of your gut microbiome, stripping away beneficial, anti-inflammatory bacteria in the small intestine and colon. This loss can damage the gut further, often paving the way for a *Leaky Gut* condition.

Furthermore, alcohol sets the stage for yeast to flourish. Having a higher tolerance to alcohol than many other microbes, yeast uses it to outcompete the beneficial bacteria in your system. This *selective pressure* is exacerbated by the yeast content of many alcoholic drinks, particularly beer. Beyond impacting the microbiome's *Composition*, alcohol's influence also extends to the microbiome's *Distribution* —even moderate drinking is associated with *SIBO (Small Intestinal Bacterial Overgrowth)*, partly because alcohol affects liver health and bile production.

Understanding alcohol's widespread role in various cultures, completely abstaining might seem impossible for some. However, during the active healing phase, excluding alcohol is crucial. I always encourage people to rethink their relationship with alcohol and consider the benefits of adopting an alcohol-free lifestyle. I made this choice when I was 22 and have never regretted it.

Take note: Occasionally, you might come across reports touting red wine's heart and overall health benefits. This demonstrates how partial truths can skew scientific facts. The real heroes behind red wine's benefits are not the alcohol but the *resveratrol* and other *polyphenols* it contains, derived from grape skins during fermentation. Let's set the record straight: these beneficial compounds aren't unique to wine; they're also found in black and red grape skins. Opting for raisins or whole grapes gives you those same benefits without alcohol's adverse effects. Note that grape juice is not a source of these potent plant chemicals because juicing doesn't involve skin extraction like winemaking does. That's why, when studies are designed to promote wine's virtues, they conveniently compare it to grape juice, sidestepping the direct comparison with whole grapes.

See also:

• Key 1 ➢ Fungi: Mold and Yeast

• Key 1 ➢ Feeding your Allies ➢ Polyphenols: The Colorful Path to a Diverse Microbiome

FOOD ADDITIVES: HACKING THE FOOD

Contrary to the toxins we discussed before, which most people try to avoid (alcohol being the notable exception), *food additives* serve a distinct purpose. Intentionally mixed into our foods, these additives are the silent partners of the food industry, designed to make products cheaper, more appealing, and longer-lasting. This shift aligns with modern taste preferences and the demand for convenience and large-scale food production.

Processed foods are teeming with additives, including:

• Preservatives extending shelf life
• Sweeteners
• Emulsifiers creating smoother textures
• Anti-caking agents preventing clumps
• Thickeners adjusting consistency

- Stabilizers keeping ingredients together
- Flavors and colors engaging our senses

Yet, these additives, like unwanted toxins, negatively impact your microbiome, liver, and the epithelial cells lining your digestive tract, ultimately affecting your immune system. As we have discussed:

> **The established safety levels for food additives and toxins disregard the selective pressure on the microbiome.**

PRESERVATIVES AND NATURAL ALTERNATIVES

For millennia, humanity had just four go-to preservatives: salt, vinegar, spices, and honey. Then sugar crashed the party in the Middle Ages as the fifth wheel. We know that too much of these, particularly sugar, can harm our health. Fast-forward to today, and the food industry has introduced an array of new preservatives that are, for the most part, much worse for our well-being.

The focus now is on cutting production costs, extending shelf lives, and ensuring that food retains its taste, smell, and texture over time. Gone are the days when we expected food stored for a long time to taste and look different, often in an unappealing way. While traditional preservation techniques prevented spoilage, they usually left food too dry, salty, or acidic. Today's preservatives and additives, however, are specifically engineered to tackle these challenges.

Nowadays, we live in a time where food's taste, smell, and texture can remain unchanged for months, even years, thanks to significant chemical interventions. This "culinary utopia" brings undeniable business benefits like lower costs, improved logistics, and market competitiveness. Yet, there's a downside. The preservatives that keep food from spoiling by killing bacteria don't discriminate; they also harm the beneficial bacteria in your gut. This creates a survival of the fittest scenario in your microbiome, favoring more resistant and potentially harmful bacterial strains over the friendlier ones, leading to decreased diversity in your gut's ecosystem.

Consider artificially hydrogenated oils and trans-fats found in numerous ready-to-eat meals and bakery products. These artificial fats are so different from natural oils that even bacteria try to sidestep them. We'll explore their impact further in Key 3, highlighting how they not only disrupt the gut microbiota but also trigger inflammation.

Your approach to preservatives should be straightforward—avoid them:

- Select raw, unprocessed foods with naturally short shelf lives.
- Avoid pre-cooked or bakery items unless they are frozen or intended to be consumed soon after preparation.
- Always check food labels for ingredients—the simpler, the better.

A few preservatives stand out as being "naturally safe and healthy" as long as they're used in moderation:

- Vinegar
- Citric acid
- Spices
- Salt (unless you have blood pressure or kidney issues)
- Honey (used infrequently)

Safe preservation techniques are:

- Freezing or refrigeration
- Drying
- Immersing in natural oil—not trans-fats
- Ozone treatment
- Brining and salting

Remember, natural preservation methods won't keep your food

fresh as long as synthetic ones do. To lengthen their effect, freeze food when needed.

See also:

• Key 3 ➤ Inflammatory Foods

• Key 1 ➤ Feeding your Allies ➤ Frozen, Dried, Salted — Preserving Raw Produce

CONCEALING POVERTY

Most food available today, except for unprocessed whole produce, is packed with food additives. Using these chemicals makes the food industry more cost-effective. Synthetic flavors cost less than their natural counterparts and sidestep the need for transportation, storage, and cleaning of raw plant-based ingredients. To illustrate, it could mean replacing truckloads of refrigerated strawberries with a single barrel of *Ethyl methylphenylglycidate*—the chemical behind that strawberry flavor. This makes the production process smoother and ensures each batch of product tastes exactly the same, regardless of the season or natural farm-to-farm variations.

Moreover, these synthetic additives allow the creation of flavor profiles that are simply unattainable with genuine natural ingredients alone. By manipulating concentrations and combining different substances, manufacturers can concoct tastes, colors, and aromas beyond what nature offers. This capacity to churn out both unique and cost-effective products secures a notable advantage in the fiercely competitive food market.

Artificial sweeteners are most concerning. As people increasingly crave sweeter tastes, amounts of these sugar substitutes are ramped up in foods, sometimes supplementing sugar or entirely replacing it in "diet" versions of junk food. But remember, swapping out sugar for artificial options doesn't transform a product into a healthier choice. Sure, added sugar is harmful, but artificial substitutes don't solve the problem.

Food additives are also used to create a variety of flavors and versions of the same product, boosting a brand's visibility on supermarket shelves. They also significantly prolong the shelf life of premade foods. Natural ingredients spoil at different rates, making fresh meals' shelf life only as long as their fastest-spoiling component. This reality doesn't work economically—vendors do not like products with short expiry times. That's why you may not find certain fresh fruits in U.S. supermarkets, like mulberries or many kinds of figs or persimmons, and why many fruits are sold unripened. Additives and preservatives keep food fresh and appealing for longer.

Another strategy manufacturers employ is adding a small amount of natural fruits or vegetables to their products, filling the rest with synthetic flavors. This move offers consumers a comforting illusion and allows labels to legally boast "made with real fruit/vegetable," even though additives shape most of the taste.

Today's food culture is often poor in whole food ingredients, with much of the diversity we see being crafted through the use of chemical additives. The focus isn't on the variety or quality of raw products, as these can be costly and less convenient for the industry. Instead, a lower-quality item is often "hacked" with additives to improve its taste, giving the illusion of quality and variety.

 When engineering cheap and tasty food, natural produce is often the least feasible ingredient to work with.

This scenario showcases the hidden nutritional poverty in prevalent modern diets, characterized by consuming lower quality and fewer varieties of products that have been engineered to disguise their taste, smell, and appearance. Imagine a time when finding added starch in sour cream would be unimaginable, yet today, it's the norm. Products are diluted, quality is compromised, and manufacturers resort to cheaper substitutes to achieve the desired texture. The challenge of finding pure, unadulterated products is increasing, as many buyers prefer more delicious "hacked" versions. Look at the yogurt section in your supermarket; the vividly flavored bottles often overshadow the traditional, plain yogurt, which might not even be available because it cannot compete. This widespread phenomenon affects nearly all 'ready-to-eat' products. Canned green peas with added sugar is another mind-boggling example. We can't fully fault companies—they merely cater to the preferences of their target markets. The decision whether or not to be part of this target group is yours.

The story of *trehalose*, a common food additive, is a telling example of how commercial interests often overshadow health considerations. Trehalose's widespread introduction to the food market around 2000 saw a corresponding rise in *Clostridium difficile* cases, a link uncovered by a study in 2018. This bacterium is associated with *Ulcerative colitis* and *Crohn's Disease*, autoimmune disorders characterized by numerous ulcers in the digestive tract. Despite this proven connection, trehalose hasn't been banned because of its value to the food industry. It's still used today, albeit in lower concentrations, to enhance the taste and texture of foods. This situation raises a critical question: What other potential hazards are hidden in our processed foods due to unnatural additives, their selective pressure on our microbiome, and their effects on various organs?

See also:

• Key 1 ≻ Food Diversity

Archaic Diet: The 1,000-Year Rule

To avoid most unnatural chemical additives, I stick to a simple rule:

 I do not eat or drink anything that did not exist a thousand years ago.

This is particularly true for products from the modern, marketing-driven food industry. Here, the race to beat the competition on price and appeal has gone hand in hand with chemical innovation. Simply put, most "processed foods" have no place on your menu.

As we discussed earlier, processed and ultra-processed items have become staples of modern diets. Shockingly, almost 60% of calories consumed in the U.S. from 2007 to 2012 were from ultra-processed foods. Not surprisingly, we're seeing a spike in microbiome and immune system diseases as well as a range of other health problems, from obesity to various cancers. Improving your health begins with a firm commitment to what I call an **"archaic diet"**—eliminating all modern, pre-packaged foods with long, technical ingredient lists.

 Buy basic whole food products and prepare your meals from scratch.

The good news is that consuming most plant-based foods raw, as previously discussed, significantly simplifies meal preparation—mostly washing, cutting, and combining. Only cook those that can't be eaten raw, like pulses.

Choose nature's simple, authentic flavors rather than the enhanced, artificial ones found in many packaged foods. Season your dishes with herbs and spices—avoid processed sauces and mixes crammed with additives. I suggest keeping a variety of dried herbs and spices at hand and using them generously to both flavor your food and support your microbiome.

Diversify your diet with a spectrum of whole plant foods rather than various kinds of brands and manufactured flavors. Shop the sections of the store that stock raw, basic produce. Venture into ethnic markets that offer a range of foods unfamiliar to the conventional Western pantry for a more diverse selection. You'll discover a richer array of whole foods in Middle Eastern, Indian, and Asian markets than in most American supermarkets. Online stores are also valuable for finding shippable items like nuts, dried fruits, herbs, spices, and seeds. Explore the world of whole foods with an open mind and creativity.

The shift begins with your approach to eating—your decision to eat whole foods, your grocery list, and how you prepare your meals. Resist letting the food industry dictate your palate with a narrow selection of chemically enhanced products masquerading as variety. Remember, YOUR preferences are YOURS to shape.

 Love the food that loves you back!

Safe Processed Food

Technically, all food preparation is a form of "processing." Yet, my caution against processed foods specifically targets methods that significantly change the food's natural chemistry or introduce chemical additives. Freezing and drying are mostly harmless unless manufacturers sneak in extra sugars or additives, so keep an eye on those labels.

Canned items? Some are fine, particularly those that are only pasteurized (heat-treated to eliminate bacteria) without additives. The same is true for single-ingredient products, like canned olives or tamarind paste, where the taste doesn't need artificial engineering because the product is merely one component of a larger recipe. These are usually a safe bet.

But, be wary of ready-to-eat meals and mixed-ingredient concoctions. They're often packed with additives to boost flavor, bypassing the need for further cooking. When shopping for packaged foods, always check the ingredient list. The shorter and simpler, the better.

Food Revolution

The 20th century witnessed many monumental societal changes and revolutions, one of which was the **Revolution of Food Culture**. After the World Wars, particularly the Second, the Western world saw a significant shift as women entered the workforce en masse. This left less time for traditional cooking, and families turned to the food industry to fill their plates.

This pivot from home-cooked meals to fast, highly processed foods has left an indelible mark on our microbiome, immune systems, and overall health. It's no coincidence that we've seen a surge in issues like obesity, metabolic syndrome, autoimmune diseases, allergies, and even cancer. The societal transformations over the last hundred years have had tangible impacts on our health. Interestingly, the microbiome is the only organ in our bodies that has undergone substantial changes during this short time.

The food industry's approach to meal preparation is worlds apart from the home-cooked practices of our great-grandmothers. It's driven by profit, focusing on reducing costs, boosting flavors, increasing addictiveness, and lengthening shelf-life. Often, achieving these goals means cutting back on natural ingredients in favor of artificial additives, as mass-produced chemicals are cheaper than their natural counterparts.

While we can't turn back the clock on the global food revolution, we can each make a stand in our own kitchens—a change you will not regret.

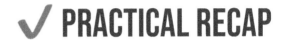

✔ PRACTICAL RECAP

DILL+ Lock: **D**ysbiosis.
5R+ Key Strategy: **R**epopulate the Microbiome.

Below are concise highlights of actionable steps for Key 1. For detailed information, please refer to the relevant chapters in this section.

- **Nutrition and Diet**
  - Enjoy fresh, traditionally made probiotic foods like fermented vegetables. Check *Bonus 2. The Art of Fermentation: Delicious Vegetable and Dairy Probiotics Recipes.*
  - Be cautious with cow's milk; sheep and goat's milk are often better tolerated. Choose fresh, traditional fermented dairy over other options. Avoid processed cheeses and dairy.
  - With few exceptions, most vegetables can and should be enjoyed raw. When needed, use mechanical processing methods. Begin with the softer, juicier varieties for easier digestion.
  - Include prebiotic foods such as fiber-rich vegetables, greens, and herbs in your diet.

- Reduce starch intake, preferably eliminating it during the active healing phase.
- Choose pulses over grains and select nutrient-rich grains over starchy vegetables and less nutritious grains. Avoid refined starchy foods.
- Eat more bitter vegetables and herbs.
- Focus on foods high in polyphenols.
- Avoid foods containing fungi—mold and yeast—like beer and other alcoholic beverages or moldy cheese.
- Sugar is your health's enemy; the same is true for both natural and artificial sweeteners. Opt for unsweetened dried fruits and non-sweet treats.
- Avoid processed foods. Avoid ready-to-eat, long shelf-life products with extensive ingredient lists.
- Ensure you're getting enough protein.
- Incorporate foods that boost the production of gastric acid, bile, and other digestive juices. When necessary, enhance your meals with acidic components to aid stomach digestion.
- Limit meat consumption, especially red meat. Opt for fish and whole plant-based foods.
- Cut out artificially hydrogenated oil, including trans-fats. Opt for polyunsaturated oils, especially omega-3-rich oils.
- Avoid artificial food additives, including sweeteners, preservatives, flavors, etc.
- Choose natural spices and herbs to enhance flavor instead of unnatural additives. Avoid spices that may irritate the gut.
- Incorporate hepatoprotective foods to support your liver health.
- Add foods with chelating properties to your diet.
- Use antimicrobial herbs and spices.

- **Holistic Nutrition Principles**
  - Make sure over half of your food intake consists of raw vegetables, fruits, nuts, and seeds.

- Love the food that loves you back!
- Do not eat or drink anything that did not exist a thousand years ago.
- When it comes to packaged foods, the simpler the list of ingredients, the better.
- Embrace food diversity. This means choosing a wide variety of basic whole-food products rather than different cooking methods.
- Shop for whole food ingredients and prepare your meals from scratch.
- Healthy food isn't a supplement to junk.
- What you eat is not just nutrients for your body; it's also the environment for your microbiota.

- **Lifestyle and Habits**
  - Prioritize natural birth and breastfeeding for your child.
  - Vegan doesn't automatically mean healthy.
  - Keep your teeth and gums healthy.
  - Refrain from eating at least four hours before bedtime.
  - Normalize body weight through healthy lifestyle choices.
  - Avoid alcohol.
  - Find effective ways to manage chronic stress.
  - Prioritize getting adequate, high-quality sleep.
  - Use special gut-flushing exercises to combat SIBO and reduce die-off reactions.
  - Practice meal spacing and periodic water fasting.
  - Thorough mastication and salivation are essential.
  - Stay well-hydrated, but remember to time your water intake wisely: drink before or a few hours after, not during meals. Also, avoid watery meals.
  - Avoid fridge-cold food and drinks.

- **Environment and Safety**
  - Ensure mold-free living and work environments, including A/C systems.
  - Use high-quality water filters to eliminate chlorine and chloramine from your drinking water.

- If using reverse osmosis filtration, add minerals back into the water to safeguard your gut epithelium from hypotonic effects.
- Opt for glass or stainless steel containers for drink storage to minimize microplastic exposure; avoid plastic bottles.
- Explore lifestyle changes as alternatives to obesity medication and bariatric surgery.
- Opt for organic foods when possible.
- Avoid consuming fish and seafood from areas known for low environmental standards.
- Opt for animal products derived from animals raised without unnatural additives, including antibiotics and hormones.
- Recognize that established safety standards for food additives and toxins overlook their selective pressure on the microbiome.
- Avoid foodborne toxins, which can stem from environmental pollution or industrial practices.

- **Supplements and Medications**
  - Incorporate supplements like Zinc, Iron, Vitamins K (paired with Vitamin D), and B_1 into your routine.
  - If necessary, consider N-Acetylcysteine (NAC) supplement.
  - Avoid antacid medications.
  - Avoid antibiotics, including those that may be present in animal products.
  - Consider using Glutathione supplements if needed.
  - For healthy bowel motility, avoid laxatives, leaning instead towards bulk-forming options, increasing hydration, and engaging in physical activities.

✚ BONUS 2. THE ART OF FERMENTATION: DELICIOUS VEGETABLE AND DAIRY PROBIOTICS RECIPES

Download the full-color, printable booklet:
https://bonus.autoimmunityunlocked.org/

Bonus 2. The Art of Fermentation: Delicious Vegetable and Dairy Probiotics Recipes

Complimentary Material for Readers

Autoimmunity Unlocked.
5 Keys to Transform Microbiome, Immune, and Digestive Health and Reclaim Your Life.
A 5R+ Holistic Guide for Rheumatoid Arthritis, Lupus, and Crohn's (Encyclopedic Edition)

Get the book at: www.autoimmunityunlocked.org

MAKE A DIFFERENCE WITH YOUR REVIEW

If you're reading this, you've already taken the first steps in transforming your health. Now, I'm asking for your help to guide others who are standing where you once stood—curious about immune health, the microbiome, and the path to reclaiming their lives but unsure where to begin.

Most people choose books based on reviews, and your words could be the encouragement someone needs to start their healing journey.

Leaving a review costs nothing and takes just a minute of your time, but the impact can ripple outward in ways you might not imagine. Simply scan the QR code or visit:

https://review.autoimmunityunlocked.org

My mission with *Autoimmunity Unlocked* is to make transforming immune health clear, accessible, and achievable for everyone.

Thank you for lending your voice to this project,

Anar R. Guliyev, M.D.
   Author

KEY 2. INFLAMMATION: REDUCE

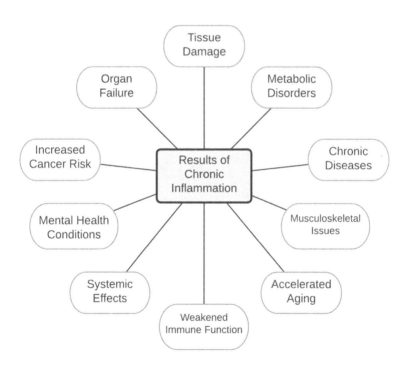

Appendix 1: Figure 4.0.2 - Chronic inflammation triggers a multitude of diseases.

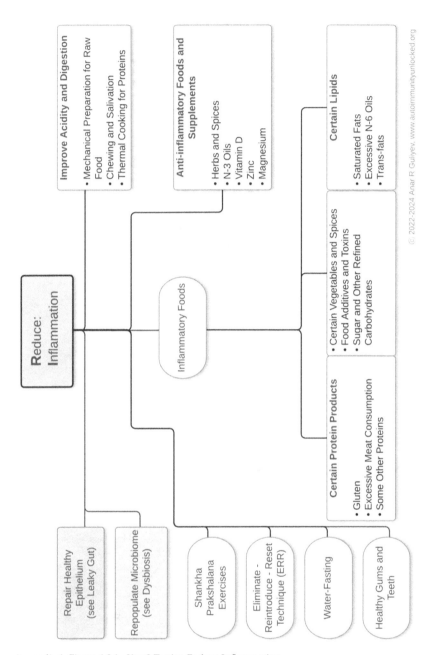

Appendix 1: Figure 4.0.1 - Key 2 Tactics. Reduce Inflammation.

INTERMITTENT HORMESIS

The timeless wisdom of "use it or lose it" is a universal truth throughout biology, affecting body and mind. Neglect exercise, and your muscles wane; start swimming or diving regularly, and your lung capacity expands; challenge your brain, and your mental agility will be preserved. Balance is key—too much of anything can tip the scale to the wrong side. Excessive physical training may lead to injuries, and trying to break records for underwater breath-holding can have even worse consequences. The concept of *hormesis* captures this delicate equilibrium.

> Hormesis is a biological phenomenon in which organs adapt and benefit from lower stress exposure that would be harmful at higher doses. The body gets stronger in response to moderate stressors and challenges.

The real takeaway, however, is that although stress magnitude must be considered, timing is more important. Our bodies and minds thrive on *intermittent stress*, followed by periods of recovery. Gym enthusiasts know that muscle growth stems from short, intense workouts followed by relaxation. This is true for every bodily function: your brain needs sleep; your heart can't endure non-stop stress; and continuous high blood pressure weakens the heart, whereas regular cardio training—

like running a few miles several times a week—strengthens it. To illustrate this concept, consider rowing: while it is a healthy sport, historically, galley-enslaved people who suffered from insufficient rest typically survived for only 3 to 4 years.

> **A chronic lack of recovery time turns even mild stressors into destructive forces.**

Months of poor nutrition damage your health, yet occasional fasting can be beneficial. Similarly, the minor annoyance of a shoe rubbing against the back of your heel—a slight, persistent, neglected friction—can lead to blisters. The same thing happens everywhere—constant, unremitting stress harms any organ.

> **Strength and resilience grow from brief periods of stress interspersed with adequate recovery intervals.**

I refer to this concept as **intermittent hormesis**, emphasizing the crucial balance between stress and recovery periods.

> The Intermittent Hormesis principle emphasizes that stress episodes must be followed by sufficient periods of restoration for hormesis to have a beneficial effect on organ health. Insufficient recovery time leads to exhaustion and degradation instead of enhanced resilience.

Understanding intermittent hormesis sheds light on addressing unhealthy gut epithelium—refer to section *Key 3: Leaky Gut*. This principle also applies to the immune system, playing a critical role in autoimmune disease development through *chronic inflammation*.

See also:

• Appendix 1 ➢ Figure 4.0.2

CHRONIC INFLAMMATION

Inflammation is often perceived as a consequence of disease, but it is a two-way street. Chronic, low-level inflammation can exhaust and harm the immune system, potentially triggering autoimmune diseases. During sickness, chronic inflammation can impede the immune system's recovery efforts, exacerbating the condition. You may have had this type of inflammation without realizing it, long before the first autoimmune symptoms surfaced.

Historically, autoimmune diseases, including arthritis, were known to be connected to chronic infections. *Rheumatic fever* is a classic example, typically associated with extended exposure to cold, damp environments and triggered by persistent *Streptococcus* infections. Similarly, many autoimmune conditions often arise following prolonged bacterial, viral, or parasitic infections.

This creates a vicious cycle: an exhausted immune system becomes inefficient against pathogens, leading to longer battles and further weakening its defenses. In some cases, the impaired immune system mistakenly begins to attack the body's own cells, triggering an autoimmune reaction. Thus, chronic inflammation wears down and derails immune cells.

You probably don't deal with extreme conditions like wading in icy water, living in damp environments, or sleeping on cold ground. And you likely overcome a common cold within a few days. However, there's a chance that a subtle, chronic inflammation could be silently affecting your immune system without your knowledge. This hidden inflammation often lurks within the digestive system, manifesting subtly as *Irritable Bowel Syndrome (IBS)* or food sensitivities. Sometimes, though, it remains undetected for years, even decades, gradually undermining your immune system's health.

See also:

• Key 1 ➤ The Many Faces of Microbiome Maldistribution: SIBO, IBS, IBD, and Ulcers

CONSEQUENCES OF CHRONIC INFLAMMATION

Chronic inflammation poses a dual threat to the immune system: *exhaustion* and *errors*. These contribute to an array of potential health issues:

- Exhausted immune system, leading to:
  - Increased susceptibility to infections
  - Heightened oncology risks
- Immune system errors, resulting in:
  - Autoimmune diseases
  - Allergies

WHEN YOU CHANGE YOUR GENES

While your genes typically remain unchanged throughout your life, there is an extraordinary exception: *lymphocytes*. These immune cells have the incredible capability to selectively alter certain parts of their DNA through a process known as *somatic hypermutation*. Their ability to change their genetic code in a controlled manner is unique, setting them apart from all other cells in your body.

Somatic hypermutation gives lymphocytes the unique ability to rewrite their DNA, tweaking their antibodies and cell receptors for a better defense. Each time they encounter a new challenge, they update their genetic code. This process of genetic fine-tuning, known as *affinity maturation*, ensures immune cells always have the best tools ready to target invaders more effectively.

> Somatic hypermutation is a cellular mechanism by which our immune system can adapt to external threats like microbes. This programmed mutation mechanism targets specific gene regions, enabling our immune cells to evolve and produce a wider range of defense molecules to counter different enemies more effectively.

Chronic inflammation transforms this unique feature into a drawback. As the immune system combats external threats, it also accidentally encounters your own cells, damaged by inflammation, toxins, and a disrupted microbiome. Over time, this constant exposure heightens the chance of harmful mutations, inaccurate affinity, and misdirected attacks. Errors in the immune response can prompt some lymphocytes to mistakenly target the body's own molecules, leading to autoimmune diseases.

These mistakes in lymphocytes' affinity maturation significantly influence autoimmune disease development. The longer the chronic inflammation lasts, the greater the chance of immune system complications. Additionally, for those already dealing with an immune system disease, chronic inflammation can worsen their condition, preventing the body's ability to eliminate defective cells and correct the issue. In short, prolonged inflammation not only increases the risk of immune system errors but also sustains and aggravates existing immune system disorders, hindering the body's ability to fix the problems.

Hence, address any signs of chronic inflammation immediately, even if it seems harmless at first glance. Inflammation, originally meant to protect your body from infections, must resolve quickly with your decisive victory, completely eliminating the threat.

IMMUNE CELLS IN THE INTESTINE

Your digestive tract exerts the greatest influence on your immune health. This significance stems from two major reasons: it's the habitat of our largest microbiome, a diverse community of bacteria, and it houses an overwhelming majority of immune cells—more than any other part of our body.

> • About 70% of our immune system's cells reside in the intestine wall.
>
> • The intestine is home to roughly 80% of your plasma cells, mostly IgA-bearing.
>
> • The gut-associated lymphoid tissue (GALT) is the body's largest immune organ.

Our digestive tract is a huge internal landscape, bigger than your skin's surface, perhaps even larger than your house. Its numerous *villi* and *crypts* form an area of 250-400 m^2 (2700-4300 sq ft). This vastness is essential for absorbing nutrients effectively but also makes it a wide-open entryway for microbial invaders. Let's be honest; the gut is far from being the cleanest part of your body. That's why it is under constant surveillance by trillions of immune cells, safeguarding this critical zone.

These "guardians of the gut" are our frontline defense against unwanted guests like pathogens and toxins. While regular quick skirmishes are normal, your built-in shield can be overwhelmed by a high number of larger, non-stop campaigns. It's important to protect these immune cells from excessive ongoing inflammatory strain. As noted earlier, chronic stress, even when subtle and unnoticed, can cause significant damage over time.

This is why much of the 5R+ program focuses on food and digestive health. Your gut's internal ecosystem is home to a vast part of both your microbiome (covered in *Key 1*) and immune system. Through *Key 2*, we aim to *Reduce Inflammation*, achieving the normal immune status of the digestive tract. Of course, this goal cannot be accomplished in isolation. All DILL+ factors are connected, and success comes only from a holistic approach involving all 5R+ Key strategies.

INFLAMMATION AND OTHER DILL+ FACTORS

Chronic inflammation of the intestine triggers a cascade of negative effects that are interconnected with other DILL+ factors.

When immune reactions are poorly regulated, they can lead to *Dysbiosis*. Certain aggressive bacteria flourish amid chronic, sluggish inflammation, outcompeting more benign ones. These pathogenic bacteria release toxins, damaging tissues and further fueling local inflammation. This sets off a vicious cycle between *Inflammation* and the *Microbiome*.

Inflammation also takes a toll on the gut epithelium, contributing to conditions like *Leaky Gut*, as we'll explore in *Key 3*. In an inflamed environment, the gut epithelium struggles to stay healthy, even when there are no other symptoms. The compromised lining becomes permeable to larger molecules, allowing them to pass through, sparking immune reactions and causing more inflammation. This sets off a vicious cycle between *Inflammation* and *Leaky Gut*, where one exacerbates the other. In severe cases, damage due to inflammation can even lead to ulcers.

In addition, inflammation damages gut nerve cells, negatively affecting intestinal motility—which we'll explore in *Key 4*. Inefficient motility leads to a buildup of toxins and bacteria, further irritating and inflaming the gut—another vicious cycle between *Inflammation* and *Lazy Gut*.

As you can see, the interaction between inflammation and the other

DILL+ factors is reciprocal: implementing all the other key strategies helps decrease inflammation, which in turn boosts their effectiveness. Focusing solely on inflammation, as many traditional and naturopathic approaches do, misses the bigger picture. This is why the results are often limited and unstable. Address all DILL+ elements simultaneously to see fundamental improvements.

See also:

• Appendix 1 ➢ Figure 4.1

DILL+ Vicious Cycles: Inflammation

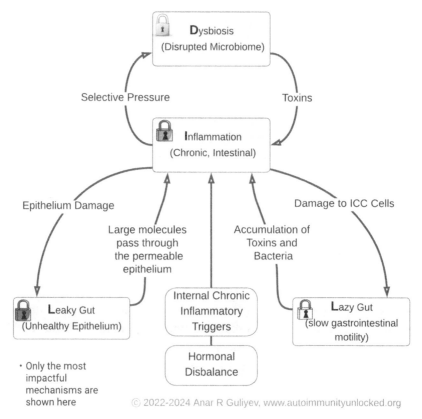

Appendix 1: Figure 4.1. DILL+ Vicious Cycles: Inflammation

INFLAMMATORY FOODS

While certain foods may trigger inflammation in the gut, not all of them are inherently unhealthy. Sometimes, even wholesome foods like nuts or berries can cause adverse immune reactions in a compromised gut ecosystem. During the recovery phase, avoid any food that worsens inflammation, given your digestive system's heightened sensitivity. However, as your gut health improves—thanks to a rebuilt microbiome, gut epithelium, and better motility (all covered by the other 5R+ Keys), along with tackling chronic inflammation—you'll be able to reintroduce a broader range of foods, even allowing for occasional indulgences.

Approach reintroductions gradually and cautiously, starting with small amounts and observing how your body responds. This careful, step-by-step process aligns with the *5R+ System's* *Reintroduce* principle. Yet, some inflammatory foods are simply unhealthy and should be avoided at all times.

FATS AND OILS

Our diet includes various fats and oils, each belonging to specific categories. For a detailed comparison, refer to Table 4.2 in Appendix 1.

Fats and Oils Cheatsheet

Type	Class	Consistency	Products
Saturated fats		solid at room temperature	• Animal-based products such as meat, dairy, and poultry. • Butter. • Coconut oil. • Palm oil.
Unsaturated fats	N-3 (omega-3) rich Oils	liquid at room temperature	• Fish. * • Flaxseed oil. • Chia seeds. • Hemp seeds. • Walnuts. • Pecans. • Canola oil **
	N-6 (omega-6) rich Oils		• Corn oil. • Soybean oil. • Sunflower oil. • Safflower oil. • Sesame oil. • Peanut oil. • Cottonseed oil. • Grapeseed oil.
	Other Oils		• Avocado oil. * • Olive oil.
Trans Fats and Hydrogenated Oils	Partially Hydrogenated (Trans Fats)	Solid or semi-solid at room temperature	• Artificially altered vegetable fats found in some processed foods. • Mostly banned in foods in the US.
	Fully Hydrogenated		• Artificially altered vegetable fats found in some processed foods.

* The highlighted categories are recommended as your primary sources of oils / fats.
** Some studies suggest canola oil may increase inflammatory markers, so it is better to avoid it.
Appendix 1: Table 4.2. Fats and Oils Cheatsheet

Our bodies require *unsaturated oils* to function optimally, while *saturated oils (fats)* aren't necessary for our metabolism. Intriguingly, both plant-derived saturated fats (like those from coconut and palm oil) and animal fats have been linked to fostering bacteria that can increase gut inflammation. So, limit your intake of saturated fats, instead opting for unsaturated vegetable oils. In particular, saturated animal fats should be avoided until you've seen significant health improvements and can benefit from *Microbiome Inertia*. This strategy also supports better heart health, mirroring the American Heart Association's recommendation to limit saturated fats to less than 10% of your daily calorie intake.

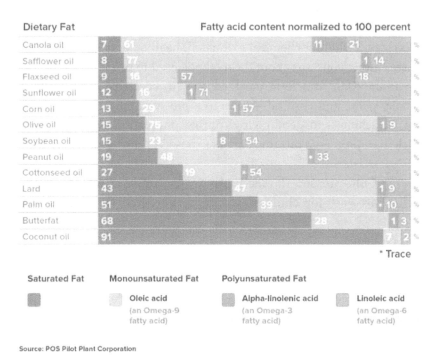

Appendix 1: Figure 4.3. Fatty Acids in some Dietary Fats

It's not just about cutting back on saturated oils; striking the right balance between unsaturated oils is also important—especially between omega-6 (N-6) and omega-3 (N-3) oils. Ideally, your diet should have an N-6 to N-3 ratio of about 3:1. But the reality for many people, thanks to the widespread use of cheap vegetable oils, is a ratio ballooning to 10:1 or even 20:1, straying far from the healthy bench-marks of the classic Mediterranean diet. This imbalance can stir up inflammation and immune system issues and also lead to broader health problems. To achieve a healthier balance, reduce the consumption of N-6-rich oils and ramp up your intake of N-3-rich oil sources like fish, nuts, seeds, and leafy greens.

Canola oil is also high in N-3 fatty acids. However, it presents a mixed bag regarding health effects. Some research suggests that heating it can create compounds that increase inflammatory markers, potentially causing harm over time. While cold-pressed might be less risky, I recommend avoiding canola oil until more conclusive research emerges. Most canola oil on the market undergoes a series of processes, including chemical extraction, heating, and refining, which raises further concerns about the methods used to produce oils.

In the U.S., the four most consumed vegetable oils—soybean, canola, palm, and corn oil—undergo a process known as RBD (refining, bleaching, and deodorizing) during production. My suggestion? Stick to unprocessed oils that are not exposed to chemical treatments.

 Cold-pressed flaxseed, olive, avocado, and walnut oils are your top choices.

See also:
• Appendix 1 ➤ Figures 4.2, 4.3

TRANS FATS AND HYDROGENATED OILS

Trans fats and processed hydrogenated oils, unlike their natural saturated and unsaturated counterparts, are seldom found in nature but have become staples in modern diets through artificial production methods. Made by transforming liquid vegetable oils into solids, foods prepared with trans fats and hydrogenated oils have a longer shelf life —even bacteria seem to avoid them. They're cheap, too, making them a favorite in the processed food industry, fast-food chains, and many diners.

But the cost to health is high. These molecules have unnatural shapes that provoke adverse reactions in our tissues. Beyond disturbing our gut microbiome, trans fats contribute to inflammation throughout the body, harming your gut, heart, and blood vessels. Despite the U.S. banning partially hydrogenated oils (trans fats) due to their undeniable links to various health issues, manufacturers can still use fully hydrogenated oils in their products. These oils, often further chemically processed (via *interesterification reactions*) to achieve certain textures, are not classified as "trans fats." While their harm seems to be lower than that of trans fats, they still present health risks, just under a different name.

Steering clear of processed foods, as recommended previously, effectively eliminates these artificially hydrogenated oils from your diet. Avoid pre-packaged meals, shortenings, margarine, spreads, bakery items, and pizzas—many of these products rely on hydrogenated oils for their preparation. This applies broadly across the spectrum, from nearly all cookies and cakes to vegan cheese and butter-like spreads, highlighting a widespread issue in the array of convenient food options available today. The traditional choice, like high-quality butter from animals raised without hormones or antibiotics, is actually healthier than these vegan surrogates. This highlights a critical point:

 Processed vegan substitutes are usually less healthy than the natural animal products they mimic.

Eicosanoids

Oils in our diet play a key role in immune health by contributing to the production of *eicosanoids*—specialized signaling molecules. These include *prostaglandins, thromboxanes, leukotrienes, lipoxins, resolvins,* and *eoxins.* These compounds regulate essential functions like inflammation, immune responses, pregnancy processes, cell growth, and blood pressure management.

Eicosanoids produced from N-6 oils tend to increase inflammation, while those from N-3 oils are anti-inflammatory. That's why getting the balance right between N-6 and N-3 oils is crucial. Interestingly, *NSAIDs (non-steroidal anti-inflammatory drugs)*, widely used in autoimmune diseases, work through the impact they have on certain eicosanoids: they inhibit prostaglandins. By changing which oils dominate your diet, you can achieve a similar anti-inflammatory result without medication.

PROTEINS AND ANIMAL PRODUCTS

When you have an unhealthy gut epithelium, also known as a *leaky gut*, eating protein-rich foods can lead to inflammation. This is because protein molecules naturally trigger immune responses. If the gut lining is compromised and lets large, partially digested protein molecules through, your immune system will react to them. This can make getting enough protein a bit tricky during treatment. That's why the foundational strategies in our 5R+ system focus on repairing the gut epithelium and restoring the population of beneficial bacteria.

Another factor that helps minimize inflammation is speeding up protein digestion. Immune reactions are mostly triggered by larger protein fragments. So, when you break down these proteins more quickly, they have less opportunity to interact with immune cells, reducing the likelihood of sensitivities. Here are a few tactics to help you do just that:

- Break down food mechanically before eating—finely chop, grind, or mill it to speed up digestion.
- Extensive heat-based cooking makes protein molecules easier to digest.
- Chew your food thoroughly to aid quicker digestion.
- Ensure your gastric acid levels and digestive processes are optimal.
- Add acidic elements like tamarind, lemon, lime juice, or vinegar to your meals to enhance protein digestion.
- Spices and herbs not only add flavor but also stimulate digestive juice production. It's best to add these after cooking so that their bioactive compounds are not destroyed by heat.

While heat-based cooking helps digest protein-rich foods, remember that most other food components, especially vegetables, are best eaten raw.

As you make progress in addressing other DILL+ factors, you'll be able to gradually increase your protein intake without the risk of inflammation.

 The faster protein molecules are broken down, the lower the risk of inflammation.

See also:
- Key 1 ➤ Stomach Acid

CHARACTERISTICS OF VARIOUS PROTEIN-RICH FOODS

- **Pulses** like lentils, chickpeas, and beans are often well-tolerated. Soak them overnight to remove *lectins*, which can cause digestive issues. Then, discard the soaking water, rinse thoroughly, cover them with fresh water, and cook them well. Kidney beans are particularly high in lectins. Wash them thoroughly, pre-soak overnight, and discard the soaking water. Rinse the beans, bring them to a boil, change the water, and boil again for 15–20 minutes. Then, reduce the heat and simmer for an additional 50–90 minutes. We will return to *lectins* in *Key 3*.
- **Fish** tends to be more gentle on the gut than meat, usually making it one of the better-tolerated protein sources. However, be mindful of potential chemical pollution.
- **Seeds**, such as pumpkin, sunflower, flax, chia, and sesame are great protein sources that are typically easily digested. Grinding most seeds aids digestion; a simple coffee grinder works well for this purpose.
- **Quinoa** - soak for 1–2 hours, then drain and rinse before covering with water to cook.

- **Nuts** are an excellent source of protein and other nutrients but may cause immune reactions due to compromised microbiota and gut epithelium. If this applies to you, consider temporarily cutting them out during the initial healing phase, then slowly reintroducing them later, carefully noting any reactions. Chestnuts are least likely to provoke a reaction, followed by almonds. Similar to seeds, grinding will aid the digestion of nuts.
- **Meat** choices matter: red meats are generally more problematic. Choose products from animals not treated with antibiotics or hormones. Pigs, cattle, and poultry often have the highest antibiotic and hormone levels, making lamb or goat better meat choices.
- **Dairy** should also be chosen with care and reintroduced only in the later stages. Select dairy from animals not treated with antibiotics or hormones. Goat or sheep milk is usually better tolerated, and fermented options are digested more easily than raw. Avoid all processed dairy, especially flavored and sweetened kinds. Cheese, due to its high protein concentration, is more likely to trigger reactions. Always avoid processed or moldy types of cheese as they are unhealthy for the microbiome. Fresh, naturally fermented probiotic dairy is the top pick. Check out the *Bonus* section for recipes.
- **Eggs** can trigger strong immune sensitivities, so usually, it's better to avoid them. If you want to reintroduce them later, choose eggs from animals that are not given antibiotics or hormones, just like you would with meat and dairy.
- **Soy-based** and other processed, artificial meat and dairy substitutes should be avoided. Whole-food pulses, nuts, and seeds are better vegan protein sources.
- **Shellfish** should generally be avoided due to its high potential for triggering immune reactions.

To check for food allergies, use the *Eliminate-Reintroduce-Reset* method (*ERR*), which will be detailed later.

To summarize, you can reduce immune reactions by mechanically breaking down and thoroughly chewing all foods. For protein-heavy foods, prolonged heat-based cooking and adding acidic elements "pre-conditions" them for faster digestion.

See also:

- Key 3 ➤ Obstacle #4: Harmful Food Ingredients ➤ Excessive Saponins and Lectins
- Key 1 ➤ Chemical Additives and Toxins in Our Food ➤ Fish Safety
- Key 3 ➤ Eliminate-Reintroduce-Reset Technique (ERR)
- Bonus 3. Food Baskets: Foods Ranked by Their Impact on the Gut-Microbiome-Immune Ecosystem.

CARBOHYDRATES

Refined carbohydrates, such as bread and pastries, and, of course, sugar, increase inflammation in the gut. As we explore more facets of a healthy lifestyle, we will see that this rule applies to many aspects:

 Always avoid sugar!

The nightshade family—including eggplants, potatoes, tomatoes, tomatillos, and all varieties of peppers—contains compounds that may trigger inflammation in those with autoimmune issues. I recommend steering clear of them during the healing phase and being cautious if reintroducing them later once the DILL+ factors have been restored.

INDIVIDUAL FOOD REACTIONS

FOOD SENSITIVITY AND ALLERGIES

About one in five Americans experience some form of food sensitivity and intolerance, where eating certain foods can trigger inflammation in the gut and other parts of the body. These conditions are often linked to a *Leaky Gut*, an unhealthy gut epithelium that allows undigested food molecules to pass through it, triggering an immune response (I will cover it in *Key 3*).

Avoiding your trigger foods can ease your symptoms but won't fix the underlying issue. The real solution is to repair the gut lining and address all the other factors of the DILL+ framework. While these repairs are underway, something that takes time, it's essential to avoid foods that trigger your sensitivities. This helps reduce inflammation and aids in restoring your digestive health and microbiome.

After restoring your gut health, a process that takes time, you can gradually reintroduce most foods into your diet—the 'Reintroduce' phase of the 5R+ system. Removing many healthy foods is usually a necessary, yet temporary step during the initial healing phase. However, you will also exclude many unhealthy foods and, hopefully, never welcome them back to your plate.

FOOD PANEL TESTS

"Food panel tests" have gained popularity lately. They check your blood for antibodies to different food ingredients to identify what you are sensitive to. However, take these tests with a big pinch of salt. Their results can be misleading, as your diet and other factors influence them.

> Many reputable organizations, like the American Academy of Allergy, Asthma & Immunology and the Canadian Society of Allergy and Clinical Immunology, advise against IgG testing for diagnosing food allergies or intolerances/sensitivities due to insufficient evidence backing its effectiveness.

These tests identify antibodies to substances that have recently come into contact with immune cells due to a leaky gut, thus sensitizing them. If you eliminate this food, its antibody levels drop, suggesting you're no longer sensitive to it. And if you start eating a new food regularly, new molecules leak through the compromised gut lining, sensitizing the immune system. This is why subsequent tests often show reactions to different products.

While these tests aren't always reliable for long-term planning, they can be valuable snapshots of what to avoid today. Think of them as a temporary map for navigating your diet's immediate no-go zones, useful for kick-starting inflammation reduction during the healing phase. Don't worry if these tests are out of reach—there are empirical ways to figure out food sensitivities through the *Elimination Diet* and the *Eliminate-Reintroduce-Reset technique,* which we'll explore in a moment. This approach requires more patience but often leads to more precise insights.

ELIMINATION DIET AND AUTOIMMUNE PROTOCOL (AIP)

The *Elimination Diet,* or *Autoimmune Protocol (AIP),* is a popular method to reduce inflammation by cutting out foods that trigger adverse immune reactions. In a nutshell, start by eliminating the usual suspects from your diet—grains, legumes, nuts, seeds, nightshade vegetables, eggs, and dairy. If symptoms persist, remove other potential triggers until you find a diet that doesn't cause inflammation. The length of this elimination phase differs from person to person and lasts until there's a significant reduction in symptoms—typically 1 to 3 months. Autoimmune responses don't switch off as quickly as food allergies. It can take several days before you notice improvements after cutting out a problematic food.

When you stop eating food that has been causing issues, the related antibody levels in your body drop, which should improve your condition. Unfortunately, the challenge doesn't end there. Many people notice that, over time, the AIP's effectiveness can wane. This happens if the foundation—the gut lining and microbiome—are not restored. When you replace eliminated foods with new ones, the molecules from these new additions will persistently leak through the compromised gut epithelium, keeping your immune cells on high alert. This ongoing sensitization means your inflammation triggers keep changing. Over time, people often find themselves having to eliminate more and more foods or frequently switching between different options to manage their symptoms. Simply removing inflammatory foods isn't enough; the underlying disease remains unnoticed like embers waiting to flare up again at the slightest provocation. The real solution involves healing your entire inner ecosystem by tackling all DILL+ factors.

Cutting out foods that fuel inflammation is still a critical step in the 5R+ system. Without it, you cannot **Repair** the intestinal epithelium, **Rouse** gut motility, or **Repopulate** the microbiome. Though, it is neither the only step nor the final one.

There are two approaches to adopting an anti-inflammatory diet:

• The traditional *Autoimmune Protocol (AIP)—top-down approach,* where you start by systematically removing sensitizing foods from your current diet, searching for the culprits until you find your optimal diet.

• The *Eliminate-Reintroduce-Reset (ERR) technique*—the *bottom-up approach,* requires more willpower and commitment but can deliver quicker, more sustainable results.

ELIMINATE-REINTRODUCE-RESET TECHNIQUE (ERR)

The ERR technique (bottom-up approach) flips the Elimination Diet on its head. Think of it as a dietary reset—beginning with an ultra-minimalist menu of foods known to be harmless, then gradually introducing new items, one by one, watching closely for any adverse reactions. Here's how it works:

1. **Start at Ground Zero:** Consider starting with a gut cleansing exercise and a few days of water fasting to effectively *Eliminate* triggers and reduce inflammation.
2. **Safe First Steps**: Kick off your dietary journey with a few carefully selected, generally well-tolerated foods. Give yourself enough time to establish a baseline of reduced inflammation.
3. **One New Product at a Time**: Gradually *Reintroduce* one new food item at a time, waiting a few days to see if any adverse reactions occur before introducing another.
4. **Backtrack When Necessary**: Should symptoms flare or inflammation increase, eliminate the last food added and give your body time to *Reset*, reducing inflammation again.
5. **Continue Moving Upward**: After the *Reset* period, cautiously add another new food to your diet, assessing your body's response.

We'll detail the plan and specific foods shortly; also check the *Food Baskets* table, where foods are categorized into several groups.

This approach enables you to progress systematically in your diet, avoiding potential inflammation triggers. From my experience, the ERR technique is more efficient and delivers quicker improvements than the AIP. By reducing inflammation in the beginning, you pave the way for your body to enhance other health aspects more effectively, laying a solid foundation for overall progress. In comparison, the classic top-down approach involves moving through inflammation while simultaneously attempting to reduce it. The ERR technique demands more self-discipline and can initially feel exasperating as you start with just a few green veggies in the early weeks.

As mentioned before, autoimmune reactions have a slow response, typically taking 6-10 days to manifest and subside. Be patient with each new food introduction, allocating sufficient time for your body to *Reset* between steps. My experience suggests that reactions during ERR unfold quicker than with AIP, with each phase lasting 2-7 days. Now, let me show you how to speed up this process even more.

See also:

• Key 4 ➢ Flushing the Gut: Ayurvedic Shankha Prakshalana Technique Simplified

• Key 3 ➢ Water-Fasting

• Appendix 1 ➢ Table 4.4

• Bonus 3. Food Baskets: Foods Ranked by Their Impact on the Gut-Microbiome-Immune Ecosystem

How to Reset Faster

The Reset step eliminates problematic foods from the gut, removes lingering sensitizing molecules from the body, and stops any inflammation that's been triggered. Initially, with an inflamed immune system, responses and recovery are sluggish.

> **The compromised immune system has a greater inertia of sickness.**

This inertia of sickness leads to delayed reactions to pathogens by an exhausted immune system and a tendency for inflammation to become chronic. Furthermore, when gut motility is slow, it takes longer to eliminate remaining food particles, extending the sensitization period. Yet, as you work on repairing the various DILL+ factors, the *Reset* process becomes faster. A healthy immune system, microbiome, and gut can regain control within a day.

Here's how to expedite the Reset phase:

Activate gut-cleansing. Eat high-fiber foods to support this process; use a *laxative* if necessary. It also helps to drink lots of water and supercharge your fiber-rich meals with olive oil. Another powerful tactic is a gut-flushing exercise routine, which we'll explore in Key 4.

Water fasting. Just one day of abstaining from food while drinking lots of water can shorten the Reset period. This helps flush out residual food particles that may ignite immune responses, cleaning both your gut and the whole body. Plus, fasting has been noted to lower inflammation levels throughout the body.

As you move forward on your healing path, you will discover that sometimes, a single day of water fasting is all it takes to hit the Reset button. This strategy can become a valuable tool in your healing toolkit. As you progress with the DILL+ factors and your general health improves, you can still experience occasional flare-ups or a resurgence of symptoms triggered by dietary missteps, infections like the common cold, or even physical exertion on arthritic joints. Interestingly, a day or two of water fasting can be just as effective as medication in helping you recover during these times.

 Hunger is a powerful weapon against inflammation.

This tactic is so effective that I strategically used it as an antidote after intentional deviations from my diet. At special events, when irresistible options were on the table, I knew I could rely on water fasting for the next day or two to offset the adverse effects of my indulgence. Of course, I strongly advise against such practice, especially during the initial healing phase. I mention this only to highlight how powerful this weapon can be, not as a recommendation for regular use.

Warning: If you're managing other health issues, particularly diabetes, water fasting may not be your best choice. In that case, a *quasi-elemental diet*, as described in *Key 3*, can be your plan B. Always consult your doctor before embarking on any fasting plan.

See also:

• Key 4 ➢ Flushing the Gut: Ayurvedic Shankha Prakshalana Technique Simplified

• Key 3 ➢ What If I Compromise My Diet? How to Reset

• Key 3 ➢ Active Repair ➢ Elemental and Semi-Elemental Diets. Quasi-Elemental Diet

Food Baskets—The Big Picture

Green Basket
(1st choice)

- Vegetables & Greens: All except hard, fibrous types and nightshade family.
- Fruits: All except those that commonly cause allergies or are high in starch.
- Vegetable Oils: Rich in omega-3 fatty acids.
- Herbs

Blue Basket
(2nd phase)

- Vegetables: All except those from the nightshade family.
- Pulses: High in protein and fiber, and easiest to digest.
- Spices: Avoid hot and irritating varieties.
- Fruits: Exclude common allergens.
- Fish

Yellow Basket
(borderline)

- Fruits: All that may cause allergic reactions.
- Grains: Only gluten-free varieties.
- Seeds
- Fermented Dairy Products: Easiest to digest and least allergenic.

Orange Basket
(minefield)

- Nuts
- Grains and Pulses
- Vegetables: Nightshade family.
- Oils and Fats: Rich in saturated fats.
- Animal Products: Non-processed cheese, meat, poultry, and eggs.

Red Basket
(avoid)

- Alcohol and Caffeine
- Artificial Additives
- Processed and Refined Foods
- Spices: Hot and irritating varieties (containing capsaicin or isothiocyanate).
- Dairy Products: Highly processed and raw milk.
- Soy Products
- Processed Meat
- Sugar
- Fats and Oils: Trans-fats and hydrogenated oils.

Appendix 1: Table 4.4. Food Baskets: The Big Picture.
For detailed lists, see Bonus 3. Food Baskets: Foods Ranked by Their Impact on the Gut-Microbiome-Immune Ecosystem

. . .

ERR JOURNEY PLAN

For an effective dietary plan, see *Bonus 3*. This guide divides foods into categories based on their impact on your microbiome, their effect on the gut epithelium, and their potential to induce inflammation. As you explore the ERR technique, tailor your diet to accommodate your body's unique immune reactions and any existing allergies. Nevertheless, this guide effectively addresses the majority of scenarios. To simplify your navigation, I've sorted foods into five 'Baskets'—*Green, Blue, Yellow, Orange*, and *Red*—starting with the Green Basket for the safest dietary options.

Start with a *Reset*, the cleansing phase discussed in the previous chapter, through water fasting, specific physical exercises, or a combination of both.

Next, select several foods from the *Green Basket* to begin your dietary journey. Expand your diet gradually, adding more Green Basket items as you progress. Stick with this Green Basket diet for a few weeks to months, depending on your body's reaction. This approach minimizes inflammation while you simultaneously apply other 5R+ strategies, laying the foundations for further improvements. Advancement within the Green Basket can be relatively swift, typically taking 1-2 days per step to check new foods.

Your nutritional journey begins with crafting a simple yet progressively enriching green salad. Start with various leafy greens and fresh herbs, then introduce energy-dense, oil-rich foods. Avocados are a good option. Next, incorporate bitter vegetables and naturally fermented foods, which are essential for your gut microbiome. To make them easier on the gut epithelium, finely chop these ingredients and mix them into salads, dressing them with flaxseed, olive, or avocado oil and a splash of lemon, lime juice, or vinegar. Also include fruits and berries from the Green Basket, opting for fresh, frozen, or naturally dried varieties, ensuring they're devoid of additives.

If your gut lining is too weak for this fiber and needs gentler food, use more mechanical preparation, like blending your salads into smoothies. I refer to this as the *Quasi-Elemental Diet*, which I will explain in more detail in Key 3.

While Green Basket foods are rich in most nutrients, they're low in protein. Yet many folks still gain lean weight and look more toned. By reducing chronic inflammation and healing the gut lining, you halt ongoing *protein loss*. This is especially true for anyone with intestinal ulcers, such as ulcerative colitis or Crohn's disease, where chronic intestinal bleeding can lead to devastating protein loss. For these patients, healing the gut lining is a game-changer. Still, we aim to progress to the next stage quickly by introducing protein-rich foods as soon as possible.

Once you're comfortable with the *Green Basket*, you can begin introducing the *Blue Basket* foods into your diet. Be cautious and take it slow, adding one food at a time and giving each new product a few days, usually 3-5, to see how you react. Be mindful of fibrous, hard vegetables that can irritate your gut lining—chopping or shredding them for salads or blending them into smoothies can make them more digestible, especially if you're managing ulcers or severe IBS. Now, you can add some protein-rich foods, starting with lentils and fish, which are generally easy on the gut. As you move forward, consider including chickpeas, quinoa, and chestnuts. Ensure to cook these protein-rich foods thoroughly, complementing them with *acidic enhancers* like lemon, vinegar, or tamarind to facilitate faster digestion.

With the Green and Blue Baskets, you already have a well-balanced, nutritious diet rich in proteins, vegetables, and oils. This is especially true if you enhance it with extra vitamin and mineral supplements from the beginning. It may feel odd to go without grains or bread, yet this diet surpasses the nutritional value of typical starch-dominated meals. It is akin to the popular *paleo diet* with an emphasis on plant-based foods. This eating style can be safely maintained for years, even decades, as you continue to work on all the DILL+ factors.

After battling rheumatoid arthritis for over 13 years, I adopted what my children humorously called the "greens-beans-fish-and-onions" diet for more than four years. Introducing new foods was daunting for me, as previous attempts often led to flare-ups. But, as my microbiome and immune cell ecosystem had restructured, I progressed rapidly with the following steps, reintroducing most of my favorite foods. Your timeline may vary—some see significant changes in months, while others, usually older adults or those with long-lasting autoimmune conditions, might need years.

Once you've built a solid foundation across all 5R+ strategies, you're ready to cautiously test the waters of the *Yellow Basket*. First, ensure your gut motility is consistently good (refer to *Key 4*). You should also have overcome other digestive issues, common indicators of an unhealthy gut epithelium and microbiome. Furthermore, it's important to be free from inflammation. Only after observing this progress over an extended period is it safe to move into the *Yellow Basket* phase. Approach this phase with extra caution, introducing new items one at a time and observing your body's response for 4-7 days. Do not rush. If you're unsure, consider a more prolonged *Reset*. Remember, you can always take several steps back or even withdraw to the safer territories of the *Green* and *Blue Baskets*.

Down the road, consider exploring the *Orange Basket*. However, remember that certain items here could be off the table for years. This applies even to perfectly healthy foods. For instance, it took me many years before I could safely reintroduce nuts to my diet. Yet, this is a small price to pay for regaining your health.

As for the *Red Basket*, rest assured you won't miss anything by permanently excluding these items.

See also:
- Appendix 1 ➤ Table 4.4
- Key 3 ➤ Quasi-Elemental Diet
- Bonus 3. Food Baskets: Foods Ranked by Their Impact on the Gut-Microbiome-Immune Ecosystem.

TRAINING WHEELS

 Both the limitations and the positive outcomes of a strict anti-inflammatory diet should be seen as temporary.

By unlocking all five DILL+ locks, you can avoid having to cut out more and more foods as sensitivities increase. Elimination diets—AIP (Autoimmune protocol) or ERR—focus only on the 'I' (Inflammation) in DILL+, never addressing the bigger picture. Unfortunately, this is a mistake I see often: people view AIP as the ultimate solution.

 Relying solely on an elimination diet is like changing only one tire when all four, plus the spare, need replacing.

But here's the upside: by thoroughly addressing all aspects through the 5R+ System, you're setting yourself up to *Reintroduce* most of the foods you've had to forego. In this sense, strict dietary restrictions act as training wheels for a beginner cyclist. They help maintain balance until your internal ecosystem is ready to master every bump and slope.

SPICES AND HERBS TO REDUCE INFLAMMATION

In addition to cutting out inflammatory foods, you can also incorporate foods that actively reduce inflammation of the gut lining. Olive oil and *N-3 (Omega-3)* rich oils are a prime example. Equally important are certain spices and herbs that quell inflammation either directly or by curbing the growth of harmful microbiota. Top choices include:

- Turmeric (Curcuma)
- Ginger
- Garlic
- Cardamom
- Oregano
- Peppermint
- Melissa (Lemon Balm)
- Rosemary
- Fennel
- Anise
- Chamomile
- Cilantro
- Basil
- Thyme
- Aloe vera

HOT OR NOT

Hot spices, especially peppers, play a notable role beyond flavor in some cultures. In India, for example, the widespread consumption of hot, pepper-rich foods isn't just about tradition or taste; it's evolved as a strategic response to the historically high risk of food and waterborne infections caused by a warm, humid climate. The strong-tasting active compounds in these spices not only block bacterial growth but also stimulate stomach acid and digestive juice production. This dual action helps combat food infections. They are also effective against conditions like *SIBO (small intestinal bacterial overgrowth)* and promote a well-balanced microbiome, thereby reducing inflammation.

However, be mindful of hot peppers, like chili, jalapeno, serrano, and cayenne. Though flavorful, they can also make the gut lining more permeable, worsen existing inflammation, and lead to new inflammation if you eat them in large amounts. For spice lovers, the drawbacks often outweigh the benefits.

Conversely, black pepper contains *piperine* instead of *capsaicin*, side-stepping any adverse effects. Swapping hot peppers for black peppers in your dishes is a safer choice, though still best used in moderation. There's a whole world of other flavorful spices for you to explore.

Spices like ginger, garlic, and onion are excellent for adding depth to your dishes while helping reduce inflammation. Conversely, mustard, horseradish, and wasabi can be harsh on your gut lining. Steer clear of these entirely, especially during the active healing phase. See also the *Cheatsheet of Inflammatory Foods and their Alternatives*.

See also:

- Key 1 ➢ Healthy Digestion to Fix Microbiota Distribution
- Key 2 ➢ Cheatsheet of Inflammatory Foods and their Alternatives
- Appendix 1 ➢ Table 4.5

SUPPLEMENTS AND INFLAMMATION

Warning: Always consult your doctor before taking any vitamins or supplements.

VITAMIN D

Vitamin D is pivotal for maintaining a robust immune system. It has powerful immunomodulatory and anti-inflammatory effects that benefit autoimmune conditions like Rheumatoid Arthritis, Lupus, and Crohn's disease. Unfortunately, people suffering from these diseases often experience profound vitamin D deficiencies. Addressing this gap through supplements can be a real game changer. Moreover, Vitamin D helps maintain healthy *testosterone* levels, which is crucial for optimal immune function.

Ideally, our bodies should get enough vitamin D from natural sunlight and a balanced diet. Yet, these sources often fall short. Our skin's ability to synthesize vitamin D decreases with age, and modern lifestyles mean we spend most of our days indoors. Additionally, those with skin conditions like lupus and psoriasis may need to minimize sun exposure, further limiting vitamin D synthesis. Herein lies another challenge: the amount of vitamin D required by an immune system exhausted from chronic inflammation is 2000-4000 IU, far exceeding the maintenance dose recommended for a healthy adult.

Vitamin D is a fat-soluble vitamin, so to ensure your body fully absorbs vitamin D supplements, consume them alongside oil-rich foods. Plus, you can amplify vitamin D's benefits by pairing it with other specific nutrients:

- **Vitamin K:** Essential for balancing calcium metabolism, which is influenced by vitamin D. For most adults, supplementing with 2000 IU of Vitamin D alongside 80 μg/day of Vitamin K is considered safe.
- **Magnesium:** Works in tandem with vitamin D to regulate immune functions. The recommended daily dose for adults is 400 mg for males and 300 mg for females.

See also:
- Key 1 ➤ Feeding your Allies ➤ Vitamin K

ZINC

Zinc has several functions in the body, making it another essential supplement for managing autoimmune diseases. Studies suggest that zinc deficiency can stimulate the production of *pro-inflammatory cytokines*, potentially disrupting immune function. Furthermore, this element plays a critical role in activating *T-lymphocytes*, and its deficiency has been linked to various autoimmune conditions.

Adequate zinc levels also support gastric acid production, which, as you may recall, is essential for a healthy microbiome. In addition, zinc is vital for wound healing, including the ongoing regeneration of the gut epithelium, meaning its deficiency can exacerbate issues like *Leaky Gut* (see *Key 3* section).

The recommended daily zinc intake varies by gender, with women needing about 9 mg and men requiring around 12 mg. Additionally, zinc aids in maintaining *testosterone* levels, a crucial hormone for immune system regulation.

See also:
- Key 3 ➤ Other Nutrients ➤ Zinc

GUM AND TEETH HEALTH

At first glance, oral health might seem unrelated. To overcome autoimmunity, though, ALL sources of chronic inflammation in your body must be eliminated. While the focus often lands on gut health, *periodontal pockets* are another common yet frequently ignored source of chronic inflammation.

> Periodontal pockets are small gaps around teeth formed when the gums recede. They are often formed due to inflammation and infection and can lead to tooth loss if left untreated.

These pockets might seem minor and are easily ignored, but seeking advice from your dentist or oral health specialist can ensure your gums and teeth remain in optimal condition. Regular dental cleanings, scaling, and, in some cases, gingival surgery might be necessary to address periodontal pockets and remove this source of chronic inflammation. We will explore this topic in detail in *Key 5*.

See also:

• Key 5 ➣ Oral Health and Other Autoimmune Triggers

CHEATSHEET OF INFLAMMATORY FOODS AND THEIR ALTERNATIVES

Table 4.5 is a cheatsheet—a concise reference guide rather than a comprehensive list. The left column contains products generally best avoided due to either adverse health impacts or their potential to exacerbate inflammation. Not all items listed are intrinsically unhealthy; some may be cautiously reintroduced into your diet after successfully fixing all DILL+ factors.

Worse	Better
Carbohydrates	
• Sugars	• Vegetables, fruits, greens, herbs—complex carbohydrates with fiber
• Refined carbohydrates	
• Synthetic sweeteners	• Resistant Starch: pulses, uncooked oats
• Refined flour	• Flatbread made from chickpea flour
• High-starch food	
• Pasta	
• Potatoes	
• Gluten-containing products and grains	
• Bread, pastry, bakery	
• Nightshade family vegetables: eggplants, peppers, potatoes, tomatoes, tomatillos	

(continued on the next page..)

Oils and Fats

- Trans-fat, hydrogenated vegetable oils—margarine, shortening, butter-like spreads.
- Deep-fried foods
- N-6 (omega-6) rich oils: corn oil, sunflower oil, safflower oil, sesame oil, peanut oil, and cottonseed oil.
- Butter
- Animal fats, lard
- Coconut oil and palm oil

- Avocado oil
- Fish oil
- Flaxseed oil
- Olive oil
- Walnut oil

Proteins and Animal Products

- Shellfish
- Red meat (beef, pork). Especially sourced from grain-fed animals.
- Meat and poultry sourced from animals treated with antibiotics or hormones.
- Processed meat
- Cow's milk products
- Dairy sourced from animals treated with antibiotics or hormones.
- Dairy with sweeteners or starch
- Raw milk
- Cheese, especially processed cheese or cheese with mold.
- Eggs
- Soy and soy products
- Peanuts and most nuts—temporary hold, until significant progress is made repairing DILL+.

- Pulses: lentils, chickpeas, and beans
- Seeds: pumpkin, sunflower, flax, chia, sesame, and quinoa
- Chestnuts
- Fish
- Other nuts—after significant progress repairing DILL+

Relatively ok alternatives:
- Lamb, goat's meat sourced from animals never treated with antibiotics or hormones—a better option than other meats.
- Naturally fermented, probiotic-rich dairy products: made of milk sourced from animals never treated with antibiotics or hormones. Free from additives. Ideally, made of sheep or goat milk.
- Some kinds of probiotic cheese. Ideally, made of sheep or goat milk. Only after significant progress repairing DILL+.

Spices and Herbs

- Mustard
- Horseradish, wasabi
- Peppers: chili, jalapeno, serrano, cayenne, etc.

- Turmeric (Curcuma)
- Ginger
- Garlic
- Onion
- Cardamom
- Aloe vera
- Anise
- Black pepper
- Herbs: oregano, peppermint, thyme, dill, melissa (Lemon Balm), rosemary, fennel, chives, etc.

(started on the previous page)
Appendix 1: Table 4.5. A Cheatsheet of Inflammatory Foods and their Alternatives

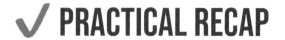 **PRACTICAL RECAP**

DILL+ Lock: **Inflammation.**
5R+ Key Strategy: **R**educe Chronic Inflammation in the Digestive System.

Below are concise highlights of actionable steps for Key 2. For detailed information, please refer to the relevant chapters in this section.

- **Food and Nutrition**
  - Avoid inflammatory foods, opting for safer alternatives. See the *Cheatsheet of Inflammatory Foods and their Alternatives* table.
  - Strive for a 3:1 ratio of N-6 to N-3 oils.
  - Thoroughly cook protein-rich foods and add acidity.
  - Use mechanical breakdown to accelerate digestion.
  - Chew food thoroughly.
  - Use spices and herbs that reduce inflammation.
- **ERR Strategy**
  - Apply the *Eliminate-Reintroduce-Reset (ERR)* technique.
  - Refer to *Bonus 3. Food Baskets: Foods Ranked by Their Impact on the Gut-Microbiome-Immune Ecosystem.*
  - Introduce protein-rich foods with great caution.

- Before reintroducing *Yellow Basket* foods, ensure you've spent sufficient time on the *Green* and *Blue Baskets*.
- Be ready to accept that some *Orange Basket* foods may be off-limits for years.
- Avoid *Red Basket* foods.
- Allow sufficient time for the *Reset* phase in ERR; if unsure, consider backing up several steps.
- Practice water fasting and special gut-flushing exercises to enhance *Resets*.

- **Oral Health**
  - Address periodontal pockets to eliminate chronic inflammation from your body.
  - Regular dental visits for cleanings and scaling are essential.

- **Supplements**
  - Consider supplements like Vitamins D, K, Magnesium, and Zinc.

- **Overall Health and Lifestyle**
  - Eliminate all chronic inflammation sources.
  - Remember: the compromised immune system has greater inertia.
  - Practice *Intermittent Hormesis*: appropriate stress followed by an adequate, proportional period of rest and restoration is necessary for all organs and systems to maintain health.
  - Remember that both the constraints and positive outcomes of an anti-inflammatory diet should be considered temporary.
  - Continue addressing other DILL+ factors even after you see improvements.

✚ BONUS 3. FOOD BASKETS: FOODS RANKED BY THEIR IMPACT ON THE GUT-MICROBIOME-IMMUNE ECOSYSTEM

Download the full-color, printable booklet:
https://bonus.autoimmunityunlocked.org/

Bonus 3. Food Baskets: Foods Ranked by Their Impact on the Gut-Microbiome-Immune Ecosystem

Complimentary Material for Readers:

Autoimmunity Unlocked:
5 Keys to Transform Microbiome, Immune, and Digestive
Health and Reclaim Your Life.
A 5R+ Holistic Guide for Rheumatoid Arthritis, Lupus, and
Crohn's (Encyclopedic Edition)

Get the book at: www.autoimmunityunlocked.org

KEY 3. LEAKY GUT: REPAIR

Though not officially recognized as a unique medical condition, the term 'leaky gut' is often used when talking about health and well-being. It refers to an *increased permeability* or 'leakiness' of the gut lining. Yet rather than an isolated issue, this 'leakiness' must be viewed as a component of a broader problem—the unhealthy state of the *intestinal epithelium*.

In the 5R+ system, I use this popular term for simplicity. However, it is important to keep sight of the bigger picture: an unhealthy intestinal lining cannot perform its functions effectively, particularly its barrier function. As with any organ in our body, its effectiveness varies, and our goal is to enhance its overall condition.

> The intestinal epithelium is a single-cell layer that forms the inner lining of the gastrointestinal tract's small and large intestines (colon). Beyond serving as a physical barrier, it plays crucial roles in nutrient absorption, secretion, and bi-directional interaction with the microbiota. Many diseases and conditions are linked to defects and dysfunctions in the intestinal epithelium.

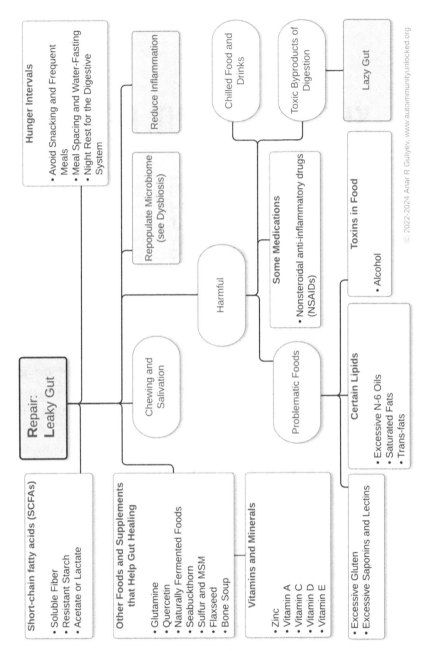

Appendix 1: Figure 5.0.1 - Key 3 Tactics. Repair Leaky Gut.

CONSTANT REPAIR

For a long time, it was thought that the first cells to perish when a person dies were brain cells. We now know this is not true. Instead, it is the cells lining the gut that succumb first. They are our 'frontline defenders'. As such, they are exposed to an aggressive environment of germs, toxins, and digestive enzymes, creating a barrier between the outside environment and our body.

Unlike our skin which has several layers, the gut epithelium is only one cell thick, making it extremely vulnerable. In addition, the lifespan of intestinal epithelial cells is surprisingly short, only 2 to 5 days. As a result, the gut lining undergoes a continuous process of renewal. Tens of billions of intestinal epithelial cells are lost and replaced daily, making the intestine one of the sites with the highest cell turnover rate in the human body.

In normal circumstances, this high regeneration rate in our digestive tract means that every 3 to 5 days, you get a brand-new gut lining. However, the story can take a different turn when the health of the epithelium is compromised—a topic I will cover in this *Key 2* section.

See also:
- Appendix 1 ➢ Table 5.1

cell type	turnover time
small intestine epithelium	2-4 days
stomach	2-9 days
blood Neutrophils	1-5 days
white blood cells Eosinophils	2-5 days
gastrointestinal colon crypt cells	3-4 days
cervix	6 days
lungs alveoli	8 days
tongue taste buds (rat)	10 days
platelets	10 days
bone osteoclasts	2 weeks
intestine Paneth cells	20 days
skin epidermis cells	10-30 days
pancreas beta cells (rat)	20-50 days
blood B cells (mouse)	4-7 weeks
trachea	1-2 months
hematopoietic stem cells	2 months
sperm (male gametes)	2 months
bone osteoblasts	3 months
red blood cells	4 months
liver hepatocyte cells	0.5-1 year
fat cells	8 years
cardiomyocytes	0.5-10% per year
central nervous system	life time
skeleton	10% per year
lens cells	life time
oocytes (female gametes)	life time

Appendix 1: Table 5.1 - Cell renewal rates in different tissues of the human body. Source: Cell Biology by the Numbers, by Rob Phillips and Ron Milo.

UNHEALTHY INTESTINAL LINING AND LEAKY GUT

Although leaky gut is not recognized as a standalone disorder, it is a well-known cause of a collection of common symptoms and health issues. For example, it is prevalent in gastrointestinal disorders such as *celiac disease*, *Crohn's disease*, and *irritable bowel syndrome*, and although the link may not be obvious, research has also revealed associations between leaky gut and many other health conditions.

When using the term 'Leaky Gut' in DILL+, I am broadly referring to an unhealthy intestinal lining or epithelium. Like any other part of your body, the gut lining can be completely healthy, very sick, or anywhere in between. As such, 'leaky gut' can manifest in many ways, thus presenting as a spectrum disorder with a wide range of potential variations.

To understand the concept of 'leaky gut', imagine a brick wall where the mortar is partially crumbling, leaving slits between some bricks. In your digestive tract, the epithelial cells in the intestine (the bricks) are held together by protein structures called *tight junctions* (the mortar). Like crumbling mortar, deficiencies in the tight junctions result in the formation of gaps between the cells, reducing the integrity of the intestinal cell wall. In addition, there might also be areas of damaged epithelium cells, ranging from microscopic spots to larger ulcers in severe cases. Fortunately, most individuals never reach this stage. However, minor structural issues with the gut lining are not uncommon. An impaired, permeable barrier is what is referred to as 'leakiness'.

The absorption of food from the intestine is a complex process controlled by the epithelial cells. In a healthy gut, only fully digested food particles are allowed to pass through the intestinal barrier. However, when this barrier function is compromised, large incompletely digested molecules, typically proteins, can make their way through the gut lining into the bloodstream where they come into contact with immune cells. As a result, an immune response may be triggered, leading to localized chronic inflammation in the gut, allergies, food intolerances, and the emergence of autoimmune processes.

However, the effects of increased gut permeability may not be immediately noticeable. Like many other chronic health conditions, low-grade issues can linger just below the surface for many years, stealthily undermining your health. The consequences are seen throughout the body and include hormonal imbalances (especially in women), chronic fatigue, fibromyalgia, skin conditions such as acne, rosacea, or eczema, and even mental health issues like depression.

Most notable, and especially relevant to this course, are the implications of 'leaky gut' for the immune system and gut microbiome. Since an increase in gut permeability doesn't occur in isolation and is associated with a range of other DILL+ factors, it is crucial to understand and address all these aspects to safeguard your health and the integrity of your body's first line of defense.

GUT LINING AND OTHER DILL+ FACTORS

A compromised gut epithelium triggers a cascade of detrimental effects that when combined with other DILL+ factors, form vicious cycles affecting your health.

Enteric toxins and large under-digested food molecules cross the compromised barrier, sparking inflammatory reactions within the intestine and potentially elsewhere in the body. This intestinal inflammation affects the nerve and muscle cells responsible for *intestinal motility*, contributing to the *Lazy Gut* condition (See *Key 4* section). Meanwhile, this local inflammation causes more damage to the epithelium, worsening leaky gut and further fueling the cycle.

Secretory cells found in a healthy gut epithelium produce (*secrete*) substances that are essential for regulating the gut microbiota. They maintain an ideal balance by killing harmful bacteria and promoting the growth of beneficial ones. When these cells are impaired, the lack of control gives rise to abnormal microbial growth and *dysbiosis*. This microbial imbalance enables pathogenic bacteria to thrive, inflicting additional damage on the epithelial cells directly, as well as through the release of toxic chemicals and inflammation. Furthermore, a decrease in the population of beneficial bacteria results in a shortfall in the amount of *short-chain fatty acids (SCFA)* they produce, which are a crucial fuel for intestinal epithelial cells (I will cover this soon). As a result, a disrupted microbiome invariably leads to an unhealthy gut lining, and vice versa.

See also:

• Key 3 ➤ Nutrition For the Gut Epithelium

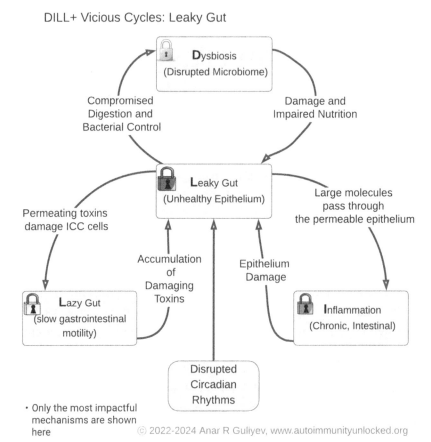

Appendix 1: Figure 5.2 - DILL+ Vicious Cycles: Leaky Gut (unhealthy intestinal epithelium)

MALABSORPTION, HYPOVITAMINOSIS, AND ANEMIA

Beyond the well-known issues of "leakiness" and inflammation, an unhealthy gut epithelium can lead to a variety of other problems, with *malabsorption* (poor nutrient absorption) being the most significant. When nutrients are not absorbed properly, people often exhibit reduced levels of vitamins and minerals in their blood, despite maintaining a nutritionally balanced diet. From my observation, the frequency of this correlation with autoimmune diseases is too high to be dismissed as a mere coincidence.

Another cause of nutrient deficiencies is an imbalance in the gut microbiota. Essentially, the overgrowth of harmful bacteria can pilfer your nutrients, resulting in a nutritional shortfall.

In addition, nutrients cannot be properly absorbed through a compromised epithelium. Nutrient absorption is not a passive diffusion of nutrients through the gut lining. Rather, it is an active process that relies on the optimal functioning of the intestinal cells. If the epithelium is unhealthy, its ability to absorb nutrients effectively declines. The unfortunate outcome is a deficiency in essential vitamins (*hypovitaminosis*) and minerals, even with a balanced diet.

To address this issue, consider "over-supplementing" your diet as you work on the root problem. Taking a good multivitamin complex and multi-mineral supplement can serve as a good starting point to at least partially compensate for poor absorption.

Repairing the gut lining and *Repopulating* the microbiome often resolve the issue, improving the body's ability to absorb nutrients. As you make headway in unlocking the DILL+ locks, you will notice significant improvements in this and other aspects of your health.

ANEMIA IN AUTOIMMUNE DISEASES

Anemia is a medical condition characterized by a decrease in the number or quality of red blood cells and a hemoglobin deficiency. These deficiencies can hinder the effective delivery of oxygen to the body's organs, leading to fatigue, weakness, shortness of breath, and even heart-related complications.

Anemia frequently accompanies autoimmune diseases as a result of the following three factors: medication side effects, intestinal bleeding, and nutrient malabsorption.

Medications such as *Azathioprine (Imuran)* and *Methotrexate* are often prescribed to suppress the immune system in conventional autoimmune treatment. However, these can also suppress blood cell production. On the other hand, our holistic, natural approach focuses on restoring a healthy immune system rather than suppressing it. By opening the DILL+ locks, the ultimate goal is to reach a stage where your doctors can confirm that you no longer need *immunosuppressants*.

Intestinal bleeding can result from ulcers or lesions. This is a leading cause of severe anemia in Crohn's and ulcerative colitis patients. However, microscopic lesions can often go unnoticed in many autoimmune diseases. The *Key 3* strategy aims to address this by Repairing the Leaky Gut and the intestinal lining in general.

Malabsorption of crucial nutrients, specifically folic acid, vitamin B_{12}, and iron, is another contributor to anemia. While you work to restore the health and absorptive function of your gut lining, it may be necessary to 'over-supplement' these nutrients. Remember to always consult your doctor about dosages. At the same time, also ensure you consume sufficient protein. As inflammation decreases and digestion improves (see *Keys 1* and *2*), so will the ability to absorb nutrients, making it easier to get enough.

Testosterone also has a role to play in blood cell production. In *Key 5*, we will work on enhancing your testosterone levels.

As you address these issues and your gut lining heals and the inflammation subsides, you should see an improvement in your blood counts. This was my personal experience—after many years of battling anemia, my levels normalized following my healing journey. In fact, this recovery has allowed me to be a regular blood donor for many years now.

See also:

• Key 5 ➢ Hormones. Why Do Females Experience More Autoimmune Conditions?

ELIMINATE OBSTACLES

Your journey to gut epithelium health encompasses two main areas: *halting the damage* and *initiating the repair*. Let's first identify the factors that damage and impair the gut lining.

 Removing harmful factors often proves more effective than adding good ones.

OBSTACLE #1: INFLAMMATION

Chronic inflammation in the intestine has a detrimental effect on the gut epithelium, even when it is low-level and otherwise undetectable. Refer to the *Key 2* section for tactics to combat this issue.

OBSTACLE #2: DYSBIOSIS

A robust microbiome is critical for the health of the gut epithelium, partly due to its production of *short-chain fatty acids*, the energy source molecules for epithelial cells. Conversely, a pathogenic microbiome can inflict extensive damage on the gut lining in multiple ways. Learn more about restoring a healthy microbiome in *Key 1*.

See also:

• Key 3 ➤ Nutrition For the Gut Epithelium

OBSTACLE #3: TOXIC BYPRODUCTS OF DIGESTION

Digestion, especially protein digestion, inherently produces toxins. This toxic load can be particularly hefty when caused by an unhealthy microbiome. For the health of your gut lining, it's crucial to efficiently eliminate these toxins, a task accomplished through active *gut motility*. The *Key 4* section provides tactics for maintaining healthy motility.

OBSTACLE #4: HARMFUL FOOD INGREDIENTS

Certain food products can be particularly taxing on the gut epithelium, making it necessary to avoid them to support the repair process. Fortunately, identifying and eliminating these items from your diet is a relatively straightforward task.

GLUTEN

> Gluten is a protein naturally found in some grains. It acts like a binder, holding food together and adding a "stretchy" quality—think of tossing and stretching out a ball of dough. Without gluten, the dough would rip easily.

In recent years, gluten has emerged as a 'problematic ingredient' in our diets, leading many to avoid it. Historically, however, gluten—a protein found in various grains—was a commonplace and nutritious component of human food. This shift raises the question: Why has gluten become problematic?

Like all proteins, gluten is meant to be digested. However, it is more difficult to digest when compared to other proteins, often remaining in the gut for extended periods. This difficulty intensifies when overall protein digestion is inefficient, a widespread issue today.

Incompletely digested gluten in the gut adversely affects epithelial cells, causing a temporary increase in gut lining permeability.

However, it typically resolves itself within 4 to 6 hours. In healthy individuals, efficient digestion reduces the duration and amount of gluten exposure, while a robust microbiome and healthy gut epithelium facilitate quicker repair, minimizing disruption. Thus, when your digestion, microbiome, and motility are all functioning optimally and inflammation is absent, the effects of gluten are minor and swiftly reversible.

Gluten-containing products	Gluten-free products
• Wheat.	Gluten-free grains:
• Barley.	• Quinoa.
• Rye.	• Buckwheat.
• Triticale.	• Rice.
• Farina.	• Millet.
• Spelt.	• Sorghum.
• Kamut.	• Oats: Choose oats that are certified gluten-free.
• Farro.	
• Couscous.	• Amaranth.
• Oats: often get contaminated during processing. Additionally, some varieties may inherently possess gluten. Opt for certified gluten-free oats.	• Corn.
	• Teff.
	Other gluten-free options:
• Soy sauce: it frequently includes wheat as an ingredient.	• Legumes: beans, peas, lentils
	• Seeds: sunflower seeds, pumpkin seeds, chia seeds, flax seeds.
	• Nuts

Appendix 1: Table 5.3 - Gluten-containing and gluten-free products

However, when any of these elements are compromised, the recovery of the gut lining can be significantly prolonged, often exceeding the time between meals. Consequently, eating another meal before complete restoration has taken place can lead to cumulative damage to the gut lining, essentially initiating a continuous cycle. Moreover, consuming gluten-rich meals less than five hours apart, even when healthy, doesn't provide enough restoration time—resulting in the same problem. And, as you may recall, increased gut permeability can expose immune cells to partially digested food molecules (including gluten), triggering inflammatory reactions and causing further damage.

Given these insights, it becomes clear that avoiding gluten is crucial during the initial stages of your health journey, particularly during the active healing stage. Once your gut health and microbiota have been restored, you may consider cautiously reintroducing gluten in small doses, if you tolerate it well. Still, ensure this is infrequent, allowing ample repair time for your gut lining between exposures. However, permanent exclusion of gluten is necessary for conditions like *Celiac disease*, *Gluten ataxia*, or other diseases with a strong reaction to gluten. Always consult your doctor before making dietary changes.

See also:

- Key 1 ➤ Stomach Acid
- Appendix 1 ➤ Table 5.3

SATURATED FATS AND EXCESSIVE OMEGA-6 OILS

When it comes to gut epithelium health, the response to different fats and oils is remarkably varied. Some oils are vitally essential, while others are harmful. As we discussed, artificially hydrogenated oils, including trans fats, increase inflammation and damage the gut lining. These should be avoided. Additionally, *saturated fats* increase the epithelium's permeability (leakiness). Therefore, I recommend limiting or excluding saturated fats during the active healing stage. Once healing is underway, you may cautiously reintroduce them in small quantities.

Research has also uncovered links between certain *unsaturated oils* and *Crohn's disease*. Consuming too much Omega-6-rich oils (N-6 oils) can increase the risk and activity of the disease. On the contrary, oils rich in Omega-3 (N-3) reduce this risk. That makes sense when considering the connection between a leaky gut and inflammation, both of which are influenced by the omega-6 to omega-3 fatty acids ratio.

Furthermore, some studies suggest that unsaturated long-chain fatty acids can increase the permeability of the gut epithelium. Conversely, *short-chain fatty acids (SCFAs)* tend to have a protective effect. This means that smaller oil molecules are typically more gut-friendly, emphasizing the importance of providing sufficient SCFAs.

So, how do we obtain these beneficial SCFAs? The answer unravels the intricate interplay between the microbiome, diet, and the gut epithelium's health: SCFAs are made in the microbiome by beneficial gut bacteria when fed with enough dietary fiber. Thus, repopulating the microbiome, consuming naturally fermented probiotic food, and following a fiber-rich diet are all crucial for your gut epithelium health.

Now consider the *low FODMAP*, meat-centric diet, often followed by people with *ulcerative colitis* and *Crohn's disease*. It involves reducing your intake of raw vegetables and increasing the amount of meat you eat. Consequently, the levels of saturated fat in your diet increase, and the amount of fiber you consume drops. While it may offer temporary relief, such a meal plan is harmful in the long run.

See also:
- Key 2 ➢ Fats and Oils
- Appendix 1 ➢ Table 4.2
- Nutrition For the Gut Epithelium

EXCESSIVE SAPONINS AND LECTINS

Saponins, Lectins, and other so-called *antinutrients* are practically unavoidable, as they are present in almost all plants. Fortunately, you don't need to avoid them entirely. The key is dosage. In small quantities, these substances can be beneficial, yet in excess, their taxing effect on the gut epithelium can do more harm.

> Saponins are a type of compound found in plants. They are often bitter-tasting and have foaming properties. Saponins can have various health effects, including lowering cholesterol, reducing inflammation, and killing bacteria. However, they can also be harmful in high doses, and they can interfere with the absorption of nutrients.

Lectins are a type of protein found in plants. They can bind to carbohydrates on the surface of cells which can have various effects, including stimulating the immune system, regulating cell growth, and promoting apoptosis (cell death). Lectins can also be harmful in high doses and can cause digestive problems.

Lectins, for example, bind directly to the lining of the small intestines. They may cause tiny lesions that contribute to the leaky gut phenomenon. Certain saponins can also increase the permeability of small intestinal cells, disrupting nutrient transport and increasing the uptake of molecules normally kept out by the gut lining. So, limit your intake, especially during the active healing stage, when you want to create optimal conditions for epithelium repair.

Several foods deserve special attention:

- **Goji berries:** These berries are one of the richest sources of dietary saponins which is why food intolerance to them is so common. If you have autoimmune conditions or food allergies, you must avoid them.
- **Soybeans:** Very high in saponins, although they are also better avoided due to their *xenoestrogen* content.
- **Other legumes:** Lentils, peas, and beans are also high in saponins and lectins. However, you can reduce the amount to safe levels by washing and pre-soaking them for several hours or overnight. The soaking water must be discarded, and the legumes rinsed before adding clean water and cooking them thoroughly.
- **Red kidney beans:** These are among the most lectin-rich foods. Wash thoroughly, pre-soak overnight, and discard the soaking water. Rinse the beans, bring them to a boil, change the water, and boil again for 15–20 minutes. Then reduce the heat and simmer for an additional 50–90 minutes.
- **Quinoa:** Soak for 1–2 hours before cooking, then drain and rinse before covering with water to cook.

- **Peanuts:** Peanuts are legumes and should be treated the same way. Presoak and cook with heat. Please note that peanut butter is still rich in lectin.
- **Nightshade vegetables:** Tomatoes, potatoes, eggplants, and peppers are high in these compounds. That's why those with autoimmune diseases often report adverse reactions to them. Avoid them during the active healing stage and reintroduce them cautiously after all DILL+ factors are restored.

Tip: When cooking pulses or quinoa, remove the whitish foam that forms on the surface. This foam is mostly made of saponins, which is why the name "saponin" originates from the same word as "soap."

With a healthy gut and a robust microbiome, you'll be well-equipped to handle these antinutrient substances, reducing the need for an extra strict diet.

See also:

• Key 5 ➤ Xenoestrogens

ALCOHOL

In earlier chapters, I described the damaging effects of alcohol on liver health and microbiome diversity. However, alcohol's harm doesn't stop there—it also damages the gut epithelium, causing inflammation and increased permeability. No level of alcohol is 'harmless.' Lower amounts simply keep damage low and less noticeable.

See also:

• Key 1 ➤ Chemical Additives and Toxins in Our Food

OBSTACLE #5: MEDICATION

Unfortunately, some common medications can also be damaging to the gut epithelium. Among these, a significant concern lies with a group known as *NSAIDs*, frequently used to treat autoimmune diseases.

Most common NSAIDs

Generic Name	Synonyms, Brand Names	Selectivity
Acetylsalicylic acid	Aspirin, ASA, Ecotrin, Aspir-Tab, Bayer Aspirin	Non-selective
Celecoxib	Celebrex, Celebra, Onsenal	Relatively more selective
Diclofenac	Voltaren, Cataflam, Dicloflex, Solaraze, Zipsor, Pennsaid, Voltaren Gel, Cambia, Flector Patch	Less selective
Etoricoxib	Arcoxia	Relatively more selective
Etodolac	Lodine, Lodine XL	Relatively more selective
Ibuprofen	Brufen, Motrin, Advil, Nuprin, Nurofen	Non-selective
Ketoprofen	Orudis, Oruvail, Actron, Ketoral, Ketoprofen Delayed-Release, Orudis KT	Non-selective
Meloxicam	Mobic, Mobicox, Arava, Vivlodex, Movalis	Less selective
Naproxen	Naprosyn, Naxen, Aleve, Anaprox, Naprosyn EC	Non-selective
Parecoxib	Dynastat	Relatively more selective

Appendix 1: Table 5.4 - Most common NSAIDs

NSAIDs

We've now reached a significant and, potentially, the most challenging hurdle in your health journey—the use of *Non-Steroidal Anti-Inflammatory Drugs (NSAIDs)*. If you have an autoimmune disease, it's highly likely you've been prescribed these medications.

> Non-steroidal anti-inflammatory drugs
> (NSAIDs) are a class of medications that are
> used to relieve pain, reduce inflammation, and
> bring down a high temperature. They are often
> used to treat symptoms of autoimmune
> diseases.

While effective in controlling inflammation, NSAIDs have an unfortunate side effect: they can damage the gut epithelium and impede its continuous regeneration. This is why ulcers and intestinal bleeding are dangerous complications of NSAID usage. Even though ulcers are rare, minor damage to the epithelium and increased permeability occur frequently. Additionally, NSAIDs can suppress beneficial bacteria, specifically *lactobacilli*, thus disrupting your microbiome.

Despite these drawbacks, you can't simply flush them down the toilet. They are essential in keeping your inflammation under control. Here lies the paradox: NSAIDs alleviate your symptoms while simultaneously contributing to the disease's underlying causes. Navigating this challenge requires collaboration with your doctor and exploring alternative routes such as the following:

- **Safer NSAIDs:** Not all NSAIDs are equally damaging to your gut epithelium. Aspirin, for instance, can be particularly harmful. However, newer generations of NSAIDs are more *selective*, thus reducing this side effect. As such, it is preferable to opt for these 'gentler-on-the-gut' selective options. See the provided Table 5.4. **Important**: Your doctor selects medication based on multiple factors. There are many other side effects to consider.
- **Topical NSAIDs:** Topical creams used for localized inflammation are safe as they don't affect the gut lining.
- **Alternative Medications:** Talk to your doctor about other classes of medication that also reduce inflammation.

Depending on your condition, they may be a viable option for you to minimize or eliminate the need for NSAIDs.

- **Anti-inflammatory Foods:** Use anti-inflammatory spices and herbs to reduce inflammation. This can help you partially or even completely replace NSAIDs.
- **Supplements:** Some supplements, like *Boswellia, Bromelain, Resveratrol*, and Vitamins D and C, can manage inflammation, helping reduce the need for NSAIDs. **Warning**: pregnant women should avoid taking *Boswellia* and *Bromelain*! Always consult your doctor about supplement use.
- **Addressing Other DILL+ Factors:** By implementing all 5R+ strategies and their tactics, you build the foundation for a healthier immune system without chronic inflammation. This allows your doctor to gradually reduce the dosage and frequency of NSAIDs, with the ultimate goal of eliminating their use altogether. But remember, this is a slow process that should be done under your doctor's supervision. To put it in military terms, NSAIDs are a fortress you cannot immediately overthrow. Instead, you need to advance on all fronts surrounding it so that this stronghold gradually loses its significance.

NSAIDs aren't limited to prescriptions for autoimmune diseases. They are also often found in over-the-counter pain relief or fever reduction medications. Frequent usage can accumulate damage in your gut, potentially triggering a vicious cycle of leaky gut syndrome, leading to further damage to your immune system. Avoid these medications whenever possible.

See also:

- Key 2 ➤ Spices and Herbs to Reduce Inflammation

OTHER MEDICATIONS

Other medical treatments, notably chemotherapy and radiotherapy, also cause damage to the gut epithelium, affecting not only gut health but immune function too. They're often a part of cancer treatment protocols, and their use typically can't be avoided. However, the fact that these treatments affect the digestive tract underscores the importance of attention to the other components of the 5R+ health system. By minimizing other harmful factors, we can help epithelium recover from such stress and support overall immunity.

OBSTACLE #6: GASTROINTESTINAL INFECTIONS

An *enteric infection*, often referred to as a stomach bug or gastrointestinal infection, can significantly disrupt your gut health. These infections are brought on by various bacteria, viruses, or parasites and can sometimes even initiate a vicious cycle toward autoimmunity.

It happens in at least three ways: a massive infection can alter your microbiome by overcoming its *natural inertia*, trigger intense inflammation, and damage the gut epithelium. This is particularly risky if you're already grappling with an autoimmune condition, making your microbiome, gut, and immune system more vulnerable. Should an infection occur during your healing journey, it can pose a significant setback. To mitigate such effects, consider the following steps:

- **Try to avoid antibiotics**. While collaborating with your doctor on treating the infection, explore the possibility of avoiding antibiotics. Often, this is achievable and beneficial in preventing further disruption to your microbiome.
- **Water Fasting**: Do a brief water fast during the infection, for 1-2 days as tolerated and under your doctor's guidance. This can prevent the leakage of large food molecules through the gut epithelium, providing time for it to regenerate.
- **Hydration**: Drink plenty of water to flush out infectious agents, toxins, and damaged cells.
- **Activated Charcoal**: Usually well-tolerated, activated charcoal aids in binding and removing toxins.
- **Gentle Diet**: During and immediately after the infection, follow a diet of light, easily digestible foods such as fruits,

leafy greens, and herbs. Include naturally fermented vegetables to help the restoration of a healthy microbiome and provide *short-chain fatty acids (SCFAs)* vital for gut epithelial health. Foods from the *Green and Blue Baskets* are best during this period.

- **Gradual Dietary Expansion**: Wait until your gut epithelium has had adequate time to heal before bringing other foods back into your diet.

Prompt and thoughtful action in response to an enteric infection can limit its impact on your health journey, helping to keep your recovery on the right path.

See also:

- Key 1 ➤ Overcoming Microbiota Inertia: Conquest or Immigration
- Key 3 ➤ Water-Fasting
- Appendix 1 ➤ Table 4.4
- Bonus 3. Food Baskets: Foods Ranked by Their Impact on the Gut-Microbiome-Immune Ecosystem.

OBSTACLE #7: INSUFFICIENT MASTICATION

Your stomach and gut epithelium, thinner than the page you're reading this on, is a delicate single-cell layer that lacks the durability to withstand the abrasiveness of numerous large food particles. Even under optimal conditions, about 100 billion gut lining cells perish and are replaced daily. Causing more of them to die may overwhelm your gut's regenerative capacity.

An excessive demand for quantity inevitably compromises quality.

Insufficient mastication (chewing) is a widespread issue in today's fast-paced world, significantly contributing to this problem. There are at least five mechanisms through which inadequate mastication can damage your gut lining.

First, mechanically. Insufficient chewing results in swallowing large pieces of food which can irritate or damage your stomach and intestinal epithelium.

These larger particles also take longer to digest as digestive juices don't penetrate them as easily. As a result, partially digested macro-molecules linger in your gut, potentially worsening 'leaky gut' conditions.

Moreover, these larger particles can serve as Trojan horses for harmful bacteria, allowing them to evade your gut's defense system of stomach acid, bile, and other digestive agents. As mentioned in *Key 1*, this affects both the microbiome and gut lining.

 Unlike lobsters, we do not have teeth in our stomachs, so take your time to chew well.

Additionally, the act of chewing stimulates other muscular activity throughout the digestive tract, thus promoting healthy *gut motility*, a topic covered in *Key 5*.

Finally, poor chewing results in less saliva being mixed with your food. Besides aiding digestion and controlling bacteria, saliva also plays a critical role in gut epithelium healing. It contains substances like *vascular endothelial growth factor (VEGF)* and *epithelial growth factor (EGF)*, which regulate the gut lining's regeneration. Insufficient supply of saliva can impair this crucial healing mechanism. Chewing involves more than the mere mechanical breakdown of food, so, regardless of how rushed you may be, do not compromise on this essential process.

Soft or semi-liquid foods often disguise the fact that this step is being bypassed. Liquid foods can move through the digestive system too quickly, leaving them only partially digested—a potential risk, especially for those with leaky gut issues. Even with the softest foods like smoothies, which I recommend for conditions such as *ulcerative colitis* or *Crohn's disease*, the act of 'chewing' and mixing food with saliva remains essential.

 Build a habit of thorough mastication—your health depends on it.

See also:
- Key 1 ➤ Mastication and Salivation — The Underrated Duo
- Key 4 ➤ Physical Activities for Optimal Bowel Transit ➤ Chewing

OBSTACLE #8: SNACKING AND FREQUENT MEALS

Every organ in our body needs downtime for restoration and regeneration. The gut epithelium is no exception. Its ongoing cycle of cell loss and replacement necessitates these rest periods.

Each time you eat, you disrupt the regeneration of your intestinal epithelium. Remember, its work is not finished at the end of a meal. It takes 2 to 5 hours for the digestive process to be complete. Only once the gut section is empty, does it have time for restoration.

Each time you reach for a snack when you feel a pang of hunger, you're denying your digestive system the rest it needs. Your stomach and gut epithelium don't get the chance to repair themselves, and your liver doesn't get to rest. This constant digestive demand results in exhausted and compromised regenerative processes (remember the concept of *intermittent hormesis*). It's one reason conditions like leaky gut and malabsorption are so prevalent today.

 Don't fear the sensation of hunger; embrace it.

Hunger stimulates the production of hormones necessary for healthy gut motility and gives your stomach, gut, and liver (which neutralizes toxins absorbed with food) a much-needed break. There are also many other beneficial processes involving hormones and metabolism, which are beyond the scope of this book.

To summarize, condition yourself to appreciate the sensation of hunger and the feeling of lightness it provides. Whether it's a short or long wait until your next meal, recognize that this period allows your body to recover. When you sit down to eat, your meal will be more enjoyable, and you'll absorb more nutrients thanks to your better-restored digestive system.

See also:

• Key 2 ➤ Intermittent Hormesis

AVOID SNACKING

The concept of snacking is relatively new. Bear in mind that for most of human history, there were no refrigerators or long-lasting packaged food. As such, snacking is a product of our modern culture, and it's not a healthy one.

In the past, despite burning significantly more calories than the modern car-driving and desk-sitting folks, our adult ancestors typically had only one to three meals a day. There was no eating outside of these mealtimes.

Interestingly, adults in some cultures, including the Turks and Mongols of the Middle Ages and the Romans before the moral downfall of their empire, practiced having just one meal a day. Apparently, they still had enough energy to create rich cultures and conquer half of the known world.

In contrast, the contemporary lifestyle avoids feelings of hunger, treating them almost as a pain that needs immediate alleviation. This mindset leads to frequent snacking, a habit far removed from the physiological norm.

 A moderate feeling of hunger throughout the day is harmless and necessary for many bodily processes.

Modern children are taught from an early age that even mild hunger must be immediately satiated. Thus begins the problem of snacking. While it's true that children should eat more frequently than adults, offering a snack to a school-aged child every few hours or whenever they feel hungry is not normal. This approach fosters bad habits, undermines discipline, and negatively affects the child's health.

MEAL FREQUENCY

As we age, our body's regenerative processes slow down, especially that of the gut epithelium. This slowdown is one reason autoimmune and other conditions often emerge as we age. Therefore, we need to give the gut more time for restoration. I recommend the following meal frequencies:

- Three meals a day for those aged 16-30.
- Two meals a day for individuals aged 30-45.
- One meal a day for those over 45.

These are general guidelines and are not cast in stone. You can add an extra meal on days you need it due to high-energy activities. However, during the active healing stage, aim to decrease meal frequency to allow more restoration time. This is necessary for the repair of your gut lining.

PLAN YOUR MEALS DIFFERENTLY

Take a more strategic approach to your meal planning to optimize intestinal epithelium restoration. Start with foods that are quickly digested like fruits and berries, then follow up with other foods about 20 minutes later. In this way, it becomes one large and lengthy meal.

Once finished, allow your digestive system to remain undisturbed. Refrain from snacking or eating anything until the next meal. This rest period, when your digestive system is "empty," is essential for the efficient restoration of the gut lining and other organs.

 Have larger but less frequent meals.

One of the tactics for giving your digestive system time to rest is *time-restricted eating*, a form of *intermittent fasting*. Here's my recommended variation:

Consume two meals within a five-hour window, having your first meal in the morning and the second meal around noon, then refrain from eating anything during the remaining 19 hours of the day. Yes, this includes abstaining from snacks. For the first meal, keep it light—consider fruits or a vegetable salad.

The second meal, closer to the end of your eating window, should be more substantial with greater protein content. The first meal digests quickly, making room for the second. The heftier second meal brings enough nutrients and calories for a day, ensuring that your digestive system will have ample restoration time until the next morning's meal.

Important: Nighttime is crucial for the rest and repair of your digestive system. As such, plan your meals to avoid eating close to nightfall.

Another effective strategy for promoting the repair of your gut epithelium is a short water fast. It involves not eating any food for a day or two, and drinking only water to ensure you stay well-hydrated. We will return to this tactic later.

Besides helping repair the gut lining, both meal spacing and water fasting can also greatly help restore a healthy microbiome.

See also:
- Key 5 ➢ Sleep and Circadian Rhythms
- Key 3 ➢ Water-Fasting

OBSTACLE #9: CHILLED FOOD AND DRINKS

When you consume chilled food and drinks straight from the refrigerator, you might not realize the harm you're inflicting on your digestive system. Here's what happens:

- **Shock to the Digestive Epithelium:** Contact with food and drinks that are too cold harms the sensitive cells lining your digestive tract.
- **Constricted Blood Vessels:** Cold temperature causes blood vessels in the stomach and gut lining to contract, hampering efficient blood circulation.
- **Slowed Digestive Juices Production:** Cold items reduce the rate at which your body produces essential digestive juices necessary for breaking down food.

- **Rapid Stomach Contractions:** The cold makes your stomach contract at a faster rate, leading to the premature passage of incompletely digested food into the intestines.

Normally, whatever you swallow should be close to your body's natural temperature.

 Don't give your stomach a temperature whiplash.

ACTIVE REPAIR

The strategy for healing an unhealthy gut epithelium is two-fold: stop the damage and start repair. Now that we've covered how to stop harming the gut lining, let's see how to repair it.

Fortunately, the gut epithelium has impressive regenerative capabilities, provided two critical resources are available: nutrition and time.

- **Nutrition:** The gut epithelium has unique energy and nutrient requirements.
- **Time:** Regeneration processes throughout the body need time. The gut epithelium is in continuous regeneration, and this process slows down when its health is compromised.

In this chapter, we'll explore the tactics within these two crucial aspects of restoring digestive health.

NUTRITION FOR THE GUT EPITHELIUM

Butyrate and Other Short Chain Fatty Acids

The health of your gut epithelium relies heavily on a few smelly substances. They are called *Short-Chain Fatty Acids (SCFAs)* and include *acetate, propionate,* and *butyrate.*

They contribute to digestive health in several ways. First, SCFAs are the primary fuel source for your intestinal epithelium. Butyrate alone provides about 70% of the energy that your gut epithelium needs to work well and heal.

Besides supplying energy, butyrate plays a critical role in synthesizing *tight-junction proteins.* These proteins are the mortar that seals the gaps between epithelial cells. Without enough butyrate, the tight junctions are compromised. This makes the gut lining more permeable, leading to the notorious *"Leaky Gut"* condition.

Moreover, SCFAs suppress many pathogenic bacteria. Thus, they help regulate your microbiome.

SCFAs deliver more health benefits, including the following:

- Stimulate blood flow to the colon.
- Enhance nutrient circulation.
- Hinder the growth of pathogens.
- Assist in mineral absorption.
- Help prevent the absorption of toxic or carcinogenic compounds.

The impact of SCFAs is so significant that butyrate supplements are used in medical treatments of the gut epithelium. You may benefit from such supplementation to jump-start the repair process in your digestive tract. Remember to always consult your doctor before starting any supplement regimen.

Butyrate supplements can be a useful tool to speed up healing. However, your goal is to restore the natural synthesis of SCFAs within your digestive system. This is a crucial function of your gut microbiome.

Factors Necessary For SCFA Production

The production of *Short-Chain Fatty Acids (SCFAs)* is driven by a healthy microbiota, which ferments fiber, especially *soluble fiber*, and *resistant starch*. Some bacteria also need small amounts of *acetate* or *lactate* to aid this fermentation. Hence, SCFA production depends on these three factors:

- Healthy Microbiota
- Soluble Fiber and Resistant Starch
- Acetate or Lactate (acetic or lactic acids)

When these three factors are lacking, the production of SCFAs is disrupted, wreaking havoc on your digestive and immune health. Your gut epithelium is starved without enough fuel. This leads to increased gut permeability, which in turn results in chronic inflammation.

As you progress with the 5R+ system, your microbiome normalizes and produces more SCFAs from the same amount of fiber. Thus, Key 1 sets up a positive momentum in your gut health journey.

SOLUBLE FIBER

Among all the essential components in your food, fiber is perhaps the most underrated. Though you don't absorb or use fiber in your body, it is critical as it nourishes your cells indirectly—via the gut bacteria.

Fiber shapes a healthy microbiome by feeding good bacteria, creating an optimal environment for them, and promoting *gut motility*. It is also vital for making *Short-Chain Fatty Acids (SCFAs)*, which are byproducts of fiber fermentation by gut bacteria. Because SCFAs are its energy source, your gut epithelium is starved without sufficient fiber. This affects its function and ability to repair itself.

Easily fermented, *soluble fiber* is particularly important for the synthesis of SCFAs. *Insoluble fiber* ferments at a much lower rate, and its function is different. We will cover more about all kinds of fiber in *Key 4*.

See also:
- Key 4 ➤ The Fiber Paradox: Why Eat What You Can't Digest
- Appendix 1 ➤ Table 6.7

. . .

RESISTANT STARCH

Earlier, we discussed starch and how it may harm your microbiome health. Unfortunately, most people's diet is largely starch-based. This widespread carbohydrate disrupts your microbiome in both dimensions:

- **Microbiome Distribution:** Like all quickly digested carbohydrates, starch skews the Microbiome population. It promotes bacterial growth in the upper part of the intestine and can contribute to SIBO.
- **Microbiome Composition:** Starch promotes the excessive growth of bacteria that prefer it for fuel. Also, it is a favorite food of yeast and mold.

One of our tactics for a healthy microbiome is to significantly reduce or even cut starch from your diet.

However, some starch molecules have a higher density and are, therefore, digested more slowly, if at all. They are known as *resistant starch*. Instead of being quickly processed in the upper intestine, they reach the lower parts of the digestive tract. As you recall, this is where the highest concentration of bacteria normally lives. Here, resistant starch functions in the same way as soluble fiber—it is fermented, and much-needed SCFAs are produced.

The best sources of resistant starch include:

- Legumes, including beans, peas, and lentils.
- Uncooked oats and barley, either rolled or cut.
- Plantains and green bananas.

See also:
- Key 1 ➢ Starch: From Protagonist to Bit Player
- Appendix 1 ➢ Table 3.11

. . .

ACETATE AND LACTATE

The third factor critical for SCFA production is the presence of *acetate* or *lactate*. Many bacteria need these acids for effective fermentation and SCFA synthesis. Normally, your gut population of *Bifidobacteria* and *Lactobacteria* make these compounds. Bacteria support each other in such symbiotic relationships—a hallmark of a healthy microbiome. If you have a disrupted microbiome, however, you may lack these types of bacteria. Fortunately, it's within your power to rectify the situation.

One simple method is adding vinegar to your food. Vinegar is mostly a solution of acetic acid in water. Sprinkle 1-2 spoons over vegetables and greens to get the necessary acetate. Naturally fermented or pickled vegetables also provide the required acidic compounds. In addition, they introduce the beneficial bacteria that produce them. This leads us to a timeless culinary tradition seen in many cultures: a salad composed of a medley of raw vegetables, greens, and herbs, flavored with vinegar or naturally fermented vegetables. The nutritional profile is further enhanced by adding vegetable oil. Use oils like flaxseed, walnut, avocado, and olive oils. These don't adversely affect your N-3 to N-6 ratios.

The same principle applies to legumes, a rich source of resistant starch. Another nod to old culinary wisdom is serving your cooked lentils or beans with a splash of vinegar or pickles. It will enhance digestion and stimulate SCFA production.

It's fascinating how modern scientific insights into gut health, the microbiome, and the immune system bring us full circle back to the traditional dietary practices of the ancient Mediterranean and Middle East.

See also:
- Key 2 ➢ Fats and Oils
- Appendix 1 ➢ Table 4.2

NATURALLY FERMENTED FOODS

Foods that undergo bacterial fermentation are already enriched with short-chain fatty acids (SCFAs). Notable examples include *turshu, sauerkraut*, *kimchi*, and a variety of other fermented vegetables. The best choice is always naturally fermented foods. Supermarket pickles are typically soaked in vinegar but lack live bacteria. They still provide some value, though, due to vinegar's acetate content, but their benefit is substantially lower.

Probiotic dairy products can also help, thanks to their lactic acid content. Cheese boasts two types of SCFAs: propionate and butyrate. Always opt for unprocessed, antibiotic-free, and hormone-free cheeses. However, if dairy products trigger food sensitivities or inflammatory reactions, especially cheese, shift your focus toward fermented vegetables instead. To learn more about fermented foods and probiotics, please refer to the *Key 1* section.

See also:

- Key 1 ➤ Probiotics
- Bonus 2: The Art of Fermentation: Delicious Vegetable and Dairy Probiotics Recipes.

OTHER NUTRIENTS

Time and again, we see specific supplements glamorized as magic potions in articles and ads. But let's be honest:

 No miracle-working superfoods can replace a lifestyle change.

To be blunt: Anyone who declares that a particular food, herb, pill, or supplement can single-handedly "fix" your issues is either delusional or lying.

Your main aim should be to address all DILL+ aspects. Eliminate damaging factors, provide nourishment to the gut lining, and rebuild your gut microbiome along with its ecosystem. When these fundamental changes are in place, some supplements, when correctly used, can offer added support. They will enhance the effectiveness of our principal strategies.

With this in mind, let's look at a few ingredients with scientifically proven benefits for gut epithelium health.

· · ·

Sᴜʟᴘʜᴜʀ ᴀɴᴅ Mᴇᴛʜʏʟsᴜʟꜰᴏɴʏʟᴍᴇᴛʜᴀɴᴇ (MSM)
Sulfur supports gut health in several ways:

- **Glutathione synthesis**: Sulfur is crucial for the synthesis of *glutathione*, a molecule previously discussed for its importance to liver health. Furthermore, glutathione is vital for tissue building and repair and is indispensable for the gut's continuous regeneration.
- **Hydrogen sulfide production**: Sulfur also contributes to the body's health through the production of *hydrogen sulfide (H_2S)*—a gas produced by the gut microbiome. It is notorious for its rotten egg smell. Yet, despite the off-putting odor, H2S is beneficial as it plays a vital role in immune regulation. A revealing study found that mice bred to produce reduced levels of H_2S had significantly fewer *T-regulatory lymphocytes*, a type of immune cell. As a result, these mice developed autoimmune diseases affecting multiple organs. This study highlights the importance of H_2S, and sulfur, in maintaining immune health.
- **Methylsulfonylmethane (MSM)**: Microorganisms in the gut lining can absorb sulfur from MSM and use it to make sulfur-containing amino acids. This positively affects the body's metabolic balance and provides nutrition to the gut epithelium.

A healthy diet provides plenty of sulfur through a variety of sulfur-rich foods such as:

- Brassicas: Cauliflower, broccoli, and leafy vegetables.
- Legumes: Chickpeas, lentils, and beans.
- Allium vegetables: Onions and garlic.

MSM and Glutathione are also available as supplements.
Important: If you have *Inflammatory Bowel Disease (IBD)*, like *ulcera-*

tive colitis or *Crohn's disease*, you may need to avoid sulfur-rich foods at first. Do this until the inflammation resolves. While sulfur is essential for a healthy gut, it can exacerbate an inflamed one. Remember to consult your doctor before making significant dietary changes or taking new supplements.

GLUTAMINE

Glutamine is your body's most abundant *amino acid* (building block of proteins). Under normal conditions, your body makes enough glutamine to meet your needs. Yet, during periods of extreme stress, such as after intense exercise or injury, you may need more glutamine than you can produce. This often happens when there is severe damage to the gut epithelium in diseases like *ulcerative colitis* or *Crohn's*.

This amino acid plays a crucial role in maintaining intestinal barrier health. Glutamine can modulate intestinal permeability and the expression of *tight junction proteins*, improving conditions like *Leaky Gut*.

Additionally, glutamine is vital for supporting your immune system function.

Dietary sources include:

- Protein-rich foods.
  - Animal products.
  - Plant-based: quinoa, lentils, beans, nuts, seeds.
- Vegetables: red cabbage, beets, dark leafy greens.

A typical diet provides 3-6 grams of glutamine daily. However, for healing purposes, the body may need much more, sometimes up to 12 grams per day. In such cases, supplements can help meet the increased demand.

Warning: Glutamine's effect on tumors is not well-studied and remains controversial. As always, consult your doctor before making any significant changes to your diet or starting supplements.

. . .

QUERCETIN

We've previously discussed the importance of *polyphenols* for microbiome health. The benefits of these potent compounds, however, extend beyond fostering a healthy microbiome. They also support digestive health and overall wellbeing.

Quercetin is a polyphenol, proven to enhance the integrity of the intestinal tight junctions. A diet rich in a variety of raw vegetables provides enough quercetin to meet your needs, making quercetin supplements unnecessary, despite their recent popularity. The following foods are rich sources of quercetin:

- Capers.
- Onions, especially the red variety, along with shallots and chives.
- Kale and broccoli.
- Various herbs.
- Berries.
- Buckwheat.
- Citrus fruits.
- Red grapes and apples, particularly the skin.
- Other brightly colored fruits and vegetables.

See also:
- Key 1 ➤ Feeding your Allies

SEA-BUCKTHORN

People have valued sea-buckthorn since ancient times. The oil from the pulp and seeds has remarkable healing properties for mucous membranes and skin as it stimulates tissue regeneration and supports the growth of healthy epithelium. For the best gut health results, eat raw fruit or oil on an empty stomach. This ensures the active components make contact with the epithelium without interference from other foods or drinks. The recommended serving is a couple of spoonfuls of oil or a handful of berries. Pills and capsules containing a droplet of oil are not efficient.

Many supplements are essentially healthy foods sold at a premium, with each bite individually packaged and priced.

Caution: Sea-buckthorn can hinder blood clotting and increase bleeding risks if you have active bleeding concerns. Always consult your doctor before consuming it.

FLAXSEED

Flaxseed alleviates irritation and inflammation of mucous membranes. It has been used since ancient times to ease stomach and gut ailments such as cramps and pain. To harness this benefit: pour hot water over ground flaxseeds; allow them to soak for a few minutes to absorb the water and form a gel-like consistency before eating it. Raw ground flaxseeds can also be added to your salad, muesli, or other food. Note, though, that whole flaxseeds are very hard. They will pass through your body undigested if you don't grind them. A coffee grinder does a fabulous job of "freeing" the nutrients of flax—or other seeds— so that you can absorb them.

Note: It's important to exercise moderation. While flaxseeds contain fewer *xenoestrogens* than soy, do not consume them daily for a long time. An occasional intake of 2-4 tablespoons is generally safe.

See also:

• Key 5 ➤ Xenoestrogens

TRADITIONAL BONE SOUP VS. BONE BROTH

You've likely heard the buzz around bone broth, often touted for its health benefits. Let's dive into this topic and unravel fact from fiction.

Bone broth has experienced an uptick in popularity, resulting in it evolving into a significant industry. While not a miracle cure, as some marketers and social media influencers claim, it does have potential dietary benefits.

Bone broth contains essential amino acids, such as proline, gluta-mine, and arginine. Although the amino acid concentration is lower than that of other protein-rich foods, a standout feature is its *bioavailability*. In other words, amino acids are easily absorbed from the broth, offering immediate benefits to the gut epithelium and microbiome. Historically, bone soup dishes were made from leftovers, especially hooves with tendons and ligaments. These usually discarded parts are also rich in *glucosamine* and *chondroitin*—compounds now recognized for joint health and often sold as supplements. Note that broth made only from bones does not contain these essential compounds.

Various cultures offer similar dishes, from Turkish *paça-çorbası* to Egyptian *kawareh* to Korean *seolleongtang*. Originally considered "food for the poor," these soups were also offered as nourishing meals for those recovering from illness.

What caught my attention was the pairing with other ingredients. Across many cuisines, these bone and tendon soups are made or served with a variety of *probiotic* and *prebiotic* foods. They include fermented vegetables, vinegar, herbs and spices like coriander, thyme, cumin, and ginger, as well as an assortment of bitter vegetables such as radishes, onion, scallions, and garlic. You may recognize these foods from the *Key 1* section, where we discussed their importance for microbiome health. It is interesting how people of different cultures empirically found healthy combinations of ingredients. Sadly, these rich traditions were largely lost when the idea was industrialized. Supermarket "bone broth" cans are mostly processed food and one more way of monetizing waste. Consider this: bone broth isn't a "drink" or "snack." Nor is it a canned supplement from a supermarket. It is a complete meal. I recommend cooking it yourself. Use whole hooves, complete with tendons, ligaments, and skin, and serve it with *probiotic* and *prebiotic* foods. As beneficial as it may be, don't make it a daily staple—it is not nutritionally balanced, and its saturated fat content is way too high.

Caution: Source these products from animals that have been raised in healthy conditions, free from antibiotics and hormones.

ZINC

Regeneration of the gut epithelium relies on various minerals. Zinc, for example, is a critical component of enzymes that are essential for protein synthesis and cell membrane structure. For this reason, tissues that grow rapidly, particularly the intestinal epithelium, heavily depend on zinc. A deficiency can disrupt this process, leading to an unhealthy gut epithelium.

Unfortunately, industrialized agriculture and soil degradation mean our food often lacks essential minerals. This is why I recommend you consider supplementing with micronutrients, including zinc. Note that men need more zinc than women.

You'll find this nutrient's importance highlighted in connection to several DILL+ factors.

See also:

• Key 2 ➤ Supplements and Inflammation ➤ Zinc

VITAMINS

Because gut epithelium regenerates quickly and has a fast metabolism, it is particularly susceptible to nutrient deficiencies. A further complication is that an unhealthy epithelium affects nutrient absorption. Also, bacterial overgrowth in the small intestine robs you of essential nourishment. As a result, you may not absorb all the vitamins your food contains. To offset this, boost the intake of micronutrients during your healing journey with supplements. Among vitamins, the most important ones to consider for our purpose are A, C, D, K, and E.

- **Vitamin A:** Vitamin A deficiency can damage the structure of the intestinal lining and impair mucus production.
- **Vitamin C**: Vitamin C is key for any regeneration and is crucial for the constant renewal of the gut epithelium. Studies also suggest it enhances microbiome diversity and promotes short-chain fatty acids production.
- **Vitamins D and K**: I've touched upon the roles of vitamins D and K in relation to microbiome health and inflammation. Both vitamins also play pivotal roles in preserving a robust

intestinal lining. Since they work hand in hand, supplement them together.

- **Vitamin E**: Vitamin E improves the gut epithelium's barrier function and mitigates inflammation. A deficiency is associated with a heightened risk of *inflammatory bowel disease (IBD)*.

By following the 5R+ dietary guidelines in this book, you will already have a higher-than-average vitamin intake. However, this may not be enough. As previously discussed, modern agricultural practices, that 'squeeze' as much as possible from the fields, mean many products nowadays are micronutrient deficient. In light of this, I recommend including vitamin and mineral supplements in your diet. As always, consult your physician to decide your optimal regimen.

See also:
- Key 1 ➤ Feeding your Allies ➤ Vitamin K
- Key 2 ➤ Supplements and Inflammation

WATER-FASTING

Besides good nutrition, every healing process demands time. During this restoration period, the healing organ should remain undisturbed. When you sustain a skin wound or a pulled muscle, you understand the importance of not aggravating it. You know that constantly scratching a wound or overstretching a hurt muscle delays recovery.

The same principle applies to your gut epithelium. A healthy gut lining regenerates quickly, often within hours. However, this rejuvenation process slows down as we age. That's why I advocate reduced meal frequency and eliminating snacking. This is beneficial even for healthy people.

In the presence of a disease characterized by an unhealthy gut epithelium, dysbiosis, and inflammation, gut healing can be very slow, requiring extra support. Water fasting is the most efficient tool to provide your digestive system with the rest it needs.

Note: In this book, "fasting" refers to water fasting for health purposes, not religious fasting that excludes water.

This method, recognized since ancient times, has been a potent remedy for many ailments. Within the framework of the 5R+ strategies, water fasting provides benefits in several ways:

- **Rest for the Gut Epithelium**: Water fasting provides a much-needed break for your gut. An *elemental diet* is often prescribed to give the gut a relative rest (a topic we'll explore in the next chapter). However, entirely abstaining from food establishes even better conditions for repair.
- **Eliminating Toxins**: The digestion of food invariably produces toxins. This is a standard process, usually well-managed by your body. Through fasting, you not only avoid introducing new toxins but also actively flush out accumulated ones with water. Unless you have a "Lazy Gut," bowel movements continue even without food. They can be enhanced by drinking plenty of water, physical activity, and special gut-flushing exercises, which we will cover in *Key 4*. Water-fasting removes toxins from both the digestive tract and bloodstream, giving the liver a well-deserved break. Altogether, this creates a better environment for gut cells.
- **Enhanced Motility**: You may be surprised to learn that in a healthy gut, hunger can stimulate bowel movements.
- **Rest for Immune System**: The gut's many chemical and biological activities keep your immune cells very busy. Fasting provides a hiatus, easing their workload in the gut. Consider how you lose your appetite when you have an infection. By reducing the digestive burden, the immune system can direct its energy toward fighting the new enemy elsewhere. This instinct proves correct—indeed, abstaining from food facilitates the healing of infections. Similarly, a refreshed immune system can better resolve chronic inflammation.
- **Reduced Inflammation and Autoimmune Reactions**: Most people report a drop in systemic autoimmune activity from the second day of fasting. For many, it feels like a big step closer to normal health. Research supports its efficacy in

conditions like IBS, IBD, rheumatoid arthritis, lupus, and other autoimmune disorders. I have already described this tactic for *Reset* in the *Eliminate-Reintroduce-Reset Technique (ERR)*. However, fasting alone is not a cure-all; it is just one tactic in our toolbox.

- **Effect on the Microbiome**: Fasting proves to be a mighty weapon against SIBO. Without a steady food supply, the bacterial population in the small intestine dwindles, and the microbes are flushed away along with their toxins.

Reduced inflammation during fasting also promotes microbiota diversity. It supports the growth of healthy microbiota, notably *Faecalibacterium prausnitzii* and *Akkermansia*. A deficiency in *Faecalibacterium prausnitzii* is associated with Crohn's disease. *Akkermansia* also offers many health benefits. It reduces inflammation, improves gut barrier function, and protects against obesity and diabetes. With this in mind, it is alarming that these bacteria have become deficient in many individuals. Notably, *Akkermansia* mainly thrives during periods of hunger.

Starting with short water fasting is simple: skip a meal or two, replacing it with large bottle of mineral water. If you've integrated the 5R+ tactic of reduced meal frequency (as discussed earlier), you're almost there. If you've transitioned to consuming just one meal a day (as I do), you're consistently practicing what's known as *intermittent fasting*. It can become second nature over time and feel quite ordinary, but it is a very effective health-promoting tool. By following such a fasting routine, you regularly give your intestinal lining most of the day to rejuvenate undisturbed.

For more substantial results, consider going a step further: skip an entire day of eating a couple of times a month. Most people find a 1-day water fast easily manageable and tolerate it well. Once you're comfortable with this, you can progress to periodic 2- and 3-day fasts. In combination with healthy eating in between, these fasts often yield significant benefits.

There are a few crucial points to bear in mind about fasting. Let's address them.

See also:

- Key 3 ➤ Obstacle #8: Snacking and Frequent Meals
- Key 4 ➤ Flushing the Gut: Ayurvedic Shankha Prakshalana Technique Simplified
  - Key 4 ➤ Water-Fasting for Active Motility
  - Key 2 ➤ Eliminate-Reintroduce-Reset Technique (ERR)
  - Key 1 ➤ Other Tactics for Fixing SIBO and Normalizing Microbiome Distribution

RULE #1: SAFETY FIRST

Always consult your doctor. Certain medical conditions may restrict your ability to fast or require a specialized regimen. For instance, the length of your fast may be limited if you have diabetes or prediabetes. For some, the *Elemental*, *Semi-Elemental*, and *Quasi-Elemental Diet*, a topic we'll explore in the next chapters, might be a more suitable alternative.

RULE #2: HYDRATION

Drinking plenty of water is essential when fasting for health. This method, distinct from religious fasting, is commonly called "water fasting." By consuming ample water, you help your body flush out toxins and any food remnants that might affect the gut lining or trigger an immune reaction. Moreover, consistent hydration supports active gut motility. Feeling hungry? Drink more mineral water.

RULE #3: PHYSICAL ACTIVITY

While you shouldn't do intense workouts while fasting, still maintain some level of activity. In other words, don't spend most of your day seated or lying down. Movement promotes intestinal motility, improves blood circulation, and aids the overall cleansing process. Even after days of water-fasting, many report having enough energy for daily tasks and a moderately active lifestyle. I recommend simple exercises such as stretches, gardening, or a stroll in the park. Always keep a positive mindset throughout.

. . .

RULE #4: GRADUAL EXIT

The importance of exiting your fast correctly cannot be over-stressed. Doing it wrong not only negates the benefits you've achieved from fasting but can also be harmful. This is especially important after extended fasting periods spanning several days. Improper exit can be dangerous. Here's the rule:

 Break your fasting gradually; the duration of your exit should be half the length of your fast.

After days of rest, your digestive system enters a dormant state. Reactivating it requires a gradual approach. It isn't just about the stomach and intestines. You must also consider the liver, endocrine functions, and your metabolism. The longer you have been hungry, the deeper the changes in your body, and the more cautious you should be switching back to your usual diet.

So, when your fasting days end, resist the urge to raid your refrigerator. Ask family members to encourage you and ensure you're on track. Plan your first post-fast meals in advance and stick to your plan. Remember, patience in progressively reintroducing food is as vital as the discipline you showed during the fast.

When transitioning back to regular eating, start with light, easily digestible foods and then gradually advance to denser, heavier ones. Visualize this progression as climbing a ladder of food "heaviness":

1. Juice
2. Smoothie
3. Whole fruit
4. Easily digestible vegetables and herbs
5. Diverse vegetables and salad
6. Legumes or grain
7. Protein-rich foods like fish and dairy
8. Meat

The longer the fast, the slower the climb. Although the type of food you eat is important, it is equally critical to eat the right amount. At each "rung" of the ladder, begin with smaller portions, then incrementally increase with each meal. Also, allow intervals for your digestive system to adapt. For example, wait at least 3-5 hours after consuming fruits or vegetables. After protein-rich foods, extend the gap even further.

This meticulous approach is crucial, especially after longer fasts where exiting might span several days. Hence, if you're new to fasting, start with a one-day fast. As you become accustomed to the practice, venture into two or three-day fasts. This brief duration makes them manageable and simpler to conclude. Here's a guideline for your exit plans:

- **1-day fast:**
  - Exit duration: Half a day.
  - First meal: Choose fruits or a small salad.
  - By your next meal, you can resume your regular diet.
- **2-day fast:**
  - Exit duration: An entire day.
  - First meal: Start with fruits or a vegetable smoothie.
  - Second meal: Switch to a green salad.
  - The following day, revert to your regular meals.
- **3-day fast:**
  - Exit duration: Two days.
  - Day one, first meal: Begin with a smoothie.
  - Day one, second meal: Transition to fruits.
  - Day two, first meal: Choose greens with herbs and oil.
  - Day two, second meal: A hearty salad.
  - By the third day, you can return to your usual healthy diet.

Tips: Adding fermented vegetables to your salad or smoothie after your fast will speed up the repopulation of your gut's microbiome. However, exercise caution if you have an active case of *Small Intestinal Bacterial Overgrowth (SIBO)*.

Also, I do not recommend any beverages besides mineral water during the fast and exit. Juices or smoothies are only suggested as first "meals" when exiting from longer fasts.

Always consult with your doctor when considering any fasting regimen.

What If I Need to Eat During Fasting?

It might seem like a paradox, but there are legitimate reasons for exceptions during a fast.

A primary concern is having to take medication. For example, it is typically not advisable to take *non-steroidal anti-inflammatory drugs* (NSAIDs) on an empty stomach. Similar guidelines apply to some other medications your physician might prescribe. In such instances, you don't have to abandon your fast altogether. Instead, opt for something light and easy on the gut, like an avocado, a fruit, or a vegetable smoothie. Your goal is to lessen the burden on your gut epithelium during this "hiatus". This approach borders the concept of the *Quasi-Elemental Diet*, which we will cover soon in the next chapter.

Some people may need to adapt the fasting protocol due to physical or psychological challenges. If, for instance, you find yourself overwhelmed by hunger or low on energy but are still determined to continue your fast, a workaround exists. A few spoons of olive oil can provide necessary sustenance without significantly disrupting the benefits of fasting. Though not an ideal method, it's a practical adjustment, especially useful for those who are just getting used to the practice of fasting.

In general, aim to keep these exceptions to a minimum to harness the benefits of fasting fully.

ELEMENTAL AND SEMI-ELEMENTAL DIETS

Water fasting provides complete rest for your intestinal lining by eliminating the need for digestion. However, you cannot survive on water alone for more than a few weeks as your body also needs a wide range of nutrients. Thus, the regime's lack of nutrition limits how long you can sustain it.

The *Elemental Diet* overcomes this problem by balancing gut rest with adequate nourishment. It replaces food with a medically formulated shake that provides easy-to-digest and readily absorbable forms of nutrients. The elemental diet is more taxing on the intestinal lining than pure water fasting. Even so, it contains all the essential nutrients, so you can continue the regimen for as long as it is needed.

Remember the importance of "restoration time"? The elemental diet allows ongoing gut repair with minimal interruptions as it optimizes eating and reduces digestive stress. Another option is the *Semi-Elemental Diet*, in which the main difference is the form of protein. In both cases, the core component is a nutrient-packed commercial shake in place of natural food.

Doctors often prescribe the elemental diet for severe gastrointestinal conditions like *ulcerative colitis* or *Crohn's disease*, especially when there's substantial intestinal damage. However, its benefits aren't limited to these ailments. Research shows that elemental diets can be as effective as *NSAIDs* or *steroid* medication for managing inflammation in many autoimmune diseases. It makes sense if we consider the link between the compromised gut lining, including Leaky Gut, and other DILL+ factors. This is why gut epithelium repair is a key strategy in our 5R+ system.

Still, I don't recommend following such a diet for the long term. Like all processed foods, elemental diet shakes may negatively affect the microbiome by decreasing its diversity. Therefore, this approach can be used short-term to promote healing, but not as a lifelong substitute for healthy whole foods.

Consult your doctor about whether the elemental or semi-elemental diet can help you kickstart the gut healing process. In the short run, it may create good initial momentum to resolve the Leaky Gut issue. However, in the long run, we want the combined benefits of other 5R+ strategies. The repopulated microbiome, reduced inflammation, and improved motility contribute to the natural healing of your intestinal lining and a return to wholesome, natural foods.

See also:

• Key 3 ➢ Obstacle #8: Snacking and Frequent Meals

QUASI-ELEMENTAL DIET

Is it possible to alleviate stress on our digestive system using natural foods? To a certain extent, the answer is yes. The primary source of irritation in the intestine is mechanical, and this is where we have some control.

My approach is an easy-to-digest diet based on the principles of the elemental diet. I call it the *Quasi-Elemental Diet*. It relies on easily digestible foods, primarily from our *Green Basket*. The key is to turn them into smoothies. Unlike commercial shakes, though, you're only breaking down the food mechanically, not chemically. Still, this is a game changer as it gives the intestinal lining a much-needed rest.

Green Basket foods are easy for the digestive system to handle, as they are devoid of complex proteins that may cause Leaky Gut reactions. They also have a low immune response profile, reducing the chances of allergies or inflammation.

Base your smoothie on either fresh vegetables or fruits. Combining fruits and vegetables in one bowl often isn't tasty. However, you can mix fruits with other fruits and vegetables with other vegetables or some other ingredients for better flavor and variety. A blender or food processor can bring your ingredients to a puree consistency to speed up digestion and minimize gut epithelium irritation.

Such a Quasi-Elemental Diet ranks after water-fasting and the *elemental diet* in creating optimal conditions for intestinal lining repair. In some ways, it is better than commercial elemental or semi-elemental products. Consuming a wide range of raw, whole, plant-based foods instead of highly processed ingredients enriches your microbiota diversity. You can take it a step further by adding *probiotic* foods to your smoothies—naturally fermented vegetables blend well with raw ones. Also, don't overlook *bitter vegetables* like garlic, onions, and ginger.

Furthermore, add herbs and spices—not only to enhance the microbiome and counter inflammation but also to improve palatability. This becomes important when you follow this regimen for many weeks. Varied food textures and the act of chewing contribute significantly to the deliciousness of our food. So, when your diet consists of homogenous purees, you have to rely more on natural flavor enhancers.

Oils are another essential component of the Quasi-Elemental Diet. Avocados work well, also prioritize olive oil and N-3-rich oils like flaxseed and walnut. They harmonize perfectly with herbs, spices, lemons, and pickles.

 Be adventurous: mix, match, and innovate.

Maintaining an adequate protein intake can be tricky on anti-inflammatory diets. One workaround is adding finely ground nuts and seeds to smoothies. In this form, they are digested faster and cause fewer problems. However, be cautious and choose only those your body has shown to tolerate well. From my experience, chia seeds, flax seeds, and cooked chestnuts are typically well-received, but monitor your body's reactions.

To further increase protein intake, consider including fish as a separate dish.

Think of your concoction as a salad transformed into a puree. If rough fiber upsets your intestines, this method ensures an adequate intake of less abrasive, ground fiber, enhancing motility without irritating the gut.

Here's what you need to remember:

- **Consistency**: Do not dilute it with water. The thicker, the better. We've previously discussed that liquid food passes too quickly through the stomach, undermining optimal digestion. If your puree turns out watery due to its fruit or vegetable content, thicken it by adding ground chia seeds, avocados, or some high-fiber ingredients.
- **Temperature**: It goes without saying, but always consume smoothies at room temperature. Chilled foods and beverages are harmful to your stomach and overall digestive health, particularly when you're in the process of repair.

- **Mastication**: Even if it's semi-liquid, chew your food. Chewing stimulates the release of saliva and promotes healthy gut motility, while saliva kickstarts digestion, controls the microbial content of food, and aids in epithelium regeneration. **Tip:** Chew gum after your pureed meal to send more saliva to your gut.
- **Alternate, do not mix**: Avoid pairing your smoothies with harder-to-digest foods in the same meal. However, you can alternate quasi-elemental meals with elemental diet shakes or a selection of healthy foods that are easy on the gut. Start with the *Green Basket*, then gradually expand to the *Blue Basket*.

The Quasi-Elemental Diet serves as a temporary yet potent tactic to enable gut lining repair until all DILL+ factors are addressed. It can be particularly beneficial for conditions like leaky gut—often seen in autoimmune cases—and more serious conditions, such as *IBS (irritable bowel syndrome)* or *IBD (inflammatory bowel disease)*. Always consult with your doctor before making significant dietary changes.

See also:

- Key 1 ➤ Actively Repopulate
- Bonus 3. Food Baskets: Foods Ranked by Their Impact on the Gut-Microbiome-Immune Ecosystem.
  - Key 4 ➤ The Fiber Paradox: Why Eat What You Can't Digest.
  - Key 1 ➤ Don't Rush the Reactor

WHAT IF I COMPROMISE MY DIET? HOW TO RESET

The potency of fasting and restorative diets on all DILL+ factors is undeniable. They form the cornerstone of your healing journey. However, there's a caveat: it's easy to be misled by the immediate, visible results they provide. Such progress, while encouraging, can be superficial, obscuring the deeper, still unresolved issues.

The most profound transformation needs to occur in your mind. Instead of simply following instructions, it is crucial first to internalize the core lifestyle principles. I often encounter people who fail to establish these foundational habits and then compromise on their diet when they notice improvements in their symptoms.

 The foundation is built in your mind, not your fridge, not even your gut.

These lapses commonly happen during social events, travels, and other similar situations. The next chapter will explore tactics to withstand these temptations. It is also vital to know how to "Reset" should you succumb.

The *Reset* process is threefold:

1. **Detoxification:** Remove the sensitizing foods you've consumed from the intestine and blood.

2. **Reducing Inflammation:** Counteract the inflammation these foods cause.

3. **Gut Repair:** Allow the gut epithelium ample time for self-repair.

Based on what we discussed previously, you can see that *water-fasting* is the best way to reset. A period without food combined with abundant hydration enables a thorough cleanse of the gut lining, promoting optimal restoration. The special exercises in Key 4 also enhance this process.

After the initial water-fasting stage, transition to gentle-on-the-gut diets like the *elemental, semi-elemental,* or *quasi-elemental.* The next step is eating only meals made with ingredients from the *Green Basket.* Also, incorporate *probiotic* foods, as any deviation from your diet that causes inflammation will likely upset your microbiome. Naturally fermented foods will help steer it back on track.

How long should the reset last? It depends. The better you have restored all 5R+ factors, the more quickly the reset will work. With a strong microbiome and motility, one day is often enough. If you're in the initial phases of the healing journey, a setback will require a lengthier reset—a few days or a week. At this stage, adhering strictly to your regimen is crucial.

The interconnectedness of DILL+ factors works against you until you unlock them—then they help you. Enhanced dynamic motility, for instance, speeds up the cleansing of your digestive system and sets up a favorable environment for beneficial bacteria. In turn, a well-established and diverse microbiome makes your internal ecosystem more resilient and adaptable, reducing its sensitivity to diet deviations. Remember the *Microbiota Inertia* principle? Finally, a sufficiently healed gut lining also regenerates faster.

I remember sometimes straying from my dietary guidelines during social events. I'd tell myself that my indulgence would be mitigated by a water fast for the next day or two. Thankfully, it worked more often than not, but it is best to avoid such lapses.

On the other hand, some people have told me this tactic was instrumental in instilling discipline. Think of it this way: if a pizza slice today means staying hungry for the entire tomorrow, you might rethink that choice. With such "dietary debt," akin to a financial one, you end up paying with interest, more than what you initially received.

See also:

• Key 4 ➢ Flushing the Gut: Ayurvedic Shankha Prakshalana Technique Simplified

• Key 2 ➢ Eliminate-Reintroduce-Reset Technique (ERR) ➢ How to Reset Faster

HOW TO AVOID TEMPTATIONS

Two tactics help uphold your dietary discipline and resist temptation:

- Replace, don't just remove.
- Come prepared.

REPLACE WITH SIMILAR PRODUCTS

When you love certain foods, simply giving them up can be challenging. Instead, swap them for similar but healthier alternatives. Here are some handy tips:

- **Sweets**: The most common craving I've observed in people is for sweets. A healthier alternative is unsweetened dried fruits.
- **Gluten-Rich Products**: For gluten-rich product alternatives, refer to Table 5.3.
- **Spicy Foods**: Hot spices can irritate the digestive system. However, some offer gut health benefits. For example, choose black pepper over red pepper.
- **Meat**: Difficult to digest, meat is one of the toughest-on-the-gut foods. Consider fish as a lighter option instead. Another well-tolerated protein source is pulses.

- For a detailed list of foods to satisfy your cravings, refer to the *Cheatsheet of Inflammatory Foods and their Alternatives* in *Appendix 1*.

 Substitute, don't exclude!

See also:
- Key 1 ➢ Sweet Does Not Equal Good
- Key 3 ➢ Obstacle #4: Harmful Food Ingredients
- Key 2 ➢ Spices and Herbs to Reduce Inflammation
- Key 2 ➢ Cheatsheet of Inflammatory Foods and their Alternatives
- Appendix 1 ➢ Tables 4.5, 5.3
- Bonus 3. Food Baskets: Foods Ranked by Their Impact on the Gut-Microbiome-Immune Ecosystem

COME PREPARED

Commitment to a diet often wavers during social gatherings or when traveling. It's common for people to rationalize indulging in off-diet foods, thinking, "It's a special occasion." Unfortunately, your health doesn't differentiate between regular days and special events. Giving in to these temptations can lead to inflammatory responses in your body afterward, creating what I refer to as an *autoimmune hangover*.

Prepare in advance if you know you are going to be in a situation where you are surrounded by tempting foods. A great strategy is eating a substantial meal before attending the event or taking your flight, as it helps fend off unhealthy cravings. While there may be some acceptable options on the menu that fall into the *Green* or *Blue Basket*, they might not suffice. By arriving with a full stomach, you enable yourself to come out as a winner—even without the self-discipline of a Navy Seal.

During my initial healing journey, I'd typically attend social gatherings already well-fed with "my food." Instead of feasting on everything, I'd scout around for one or two suitable items. Most main courses contain numerous ingredients, and not all of them are healthy.

They may include undesirable oils and many dishes are starch-heavy —a no-no when aiming to restore the microbiome. Yet, there can be side offerings like fresh veggies, olives, pickles, and fruits. Drinks can also be a little tricky. Natural juices are a good choice (not nectars and other sugary "juice-like drinks"), but mineral water often stands out as the only healthy beverage option available at social gatherings. Filling your belly with healthy food before an event is empowering, making it easy to be very picky.

When I expect a dessert-heavy gathering, I offer a contribution to the meal. I bring along natural sweet treats, like fresh or dried fruits and nuts. It allows me to enjoy my whole-food sweets while others, unfortunately, choose to poison themselves with cake or ice cream. These are no longer a temptation for me—I do not perceive man-made desserts as food. Being proactive in such cases means I don't have to go hungry. Interestingly, what I bring is often appreciated by other guests who acknowledge the benefits of healthy treats. Hence, I always pack plenty, ensuring there's enough to share.

This tactic is straightforward to implement. When out and about, consider packing dried fruits with nuts or seeds. These nutrient-dense, non-perishable items need neither preparation nor refrigeration, making them especially handy while traveling.

✔ PRACTICAL RECAP

DILL+ Lock: Leaky gut.
5R+ Key Strategy: **R**epair Healthy Gut Epithelium.

Below are concise highlights of actionable steps for Key 3. For detailed information, please refer to the relevant chapters in this section.

- **Dietary Recommendations:**
  - Avoid:
    - Gluten
    - Trans fats and artificially hydrogenated oils
    - Excessive saturated fats
    - Excessive N-6 oils
    - Excessive saponins and lectins
    - Alcohol
  - Increase:
    - Proportions of N-3 oils
    - Naturally fermented foods
    - For SCFA Synthesis:
      - Soluble fiber
      - Resistant starch
      - Acetate or lactate
- **Specific Foods and Supplements:**

- ◦ Glutamine
- ◦ Quercetin
- ◦ Zinc
- ◦ Vitamins A, C, D, K, and E
- ◦ Flaxseed and sea-buckthorn
- ◦ Sulfur and methylsulfonylmethane (MSM)
- **Eating Habits:**
  - ◦ Avoid chilled foods and drinks
  - ◦ Avoid snacking and reduce meal frequency
  - ◦ Build a habit of thorough mastication and salivation
  - ◦ Practice time-restricted eating and meal spacing
  - ◦ Ensure night rest for the digestive system
- **Dietary Interventions:**
  - ◦ Water fasting
  - ◦ Elemental and semi-elemental diets
  - ◦ Quasi-elemental diet
  - ◦ *Reset* if the diet was compromised
- **Tips for Adherence:**
  - ◦ Substitute, don't exclude!
  - ◦ Come prepared
- **Mitigate the effects of NSAID medications**

KEY 4. LAZY GUT: REAWAKEN

Advertisements for home water filters stress the hidden risks of toxic buildup in your property's plumbing. They show how their filtration systems trap various impurities, from chemicals to pathogens. Indeed, it is quite unsettling to consider what might be lurking in your tap water. Unfortunately, many people live with contaminated pipes—not in the kitchen but within their own bodies.

Your alimentary system's main tasks are digestion and nutrient absorption. It is also the biggest immune hub in your body and the largest surface where your blood nearly meets the dangers of the outside world. It is very resilient and adaptable. Yet, it is not meant to be a storage facility for toxins, rotting waste, mold, parasites, and harmful infections.

We've discussed how the internal environment shapes our microbiome and immune cell population. Besides food, a vital aspect of a healthy digestive system is how efficiently it moves its contents—its motility. Effective intestinal motion prevents stagnation and the buildup of harmful pathogens.

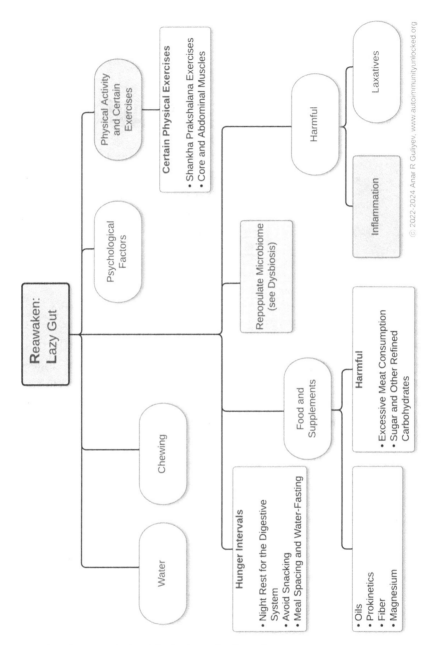

Appendix 1: Figure 6.0.1 - Key 4 Tactics. Reawaken Lazy Gut.

GUT MOTILITY: SPEEDY OR SLUGGISH

HEALTHY MOTILITY

Gastrointestinal (GI) Motility is the term used for the muscle contractions that propel food through the digestive system. The synchronized contractions of these muscles are called peristalsis. These controlled movements ensure the contents of the digestive tract move in one direction and at a consistent pace. Simultaneously, they enable the absorption of essential nutrients and the removal of digestive by-products and toxins. In addition, gut motility regulates the colonization of the microbial ecosystem (microbiome).

Did you know you can eat while hanging upside down, and your food will still travel in the right direction? This is due to *peristalsis*, wave-like motions generated by the muscles of your alimentary canal. They ensure food moves in one direction at a consistent pace throughout your digestive tract.

This movement is so essential to life that it operates on autopilot. Just as your heart beats without you having to think about it, your digestive system functions without the brain's direct intervention. Few bodily movements can boast this level of self-governance.

To make it possible, your gut has a unique *enteric nervous system*, often called the "second brain." It is the largest collection of neurons outside the central nervous system (your brain and spinal cord). Nestled within the walls of the digestive tract, it oversees gut reflexes. Thus, managing gastrointestinal motility (movement), blood flow, and fluid transport.

LAZY GUT CONDITION

When I refer to a "Lazy Gut," I'm talking about gut motility that is slower and less active than it should be. The increased time it takes for contents to pass through the intestines results in less frequent bowel movements. Though, it is not a full-blown constipation.

How often should you have a bowel movement? The answer varies based on several factors. Here is a simple guideline: as frequent as your meals, or a bit more. Picture it like traffic: if you're taking in food twice daily but only expelling waste once, you create a traffic jam. The mismatch between intake and bowel evacuation suggests stagnation within your system.

I know that medical standards for bowel movements have shifted. For this reason, some now claim that evacuating as infrequently as four times a week is "normal." It is not. It has just become common.

 Common does not mean normal!

BOWEL TRANSIT TIME

The frequency of bowel movements only tells part of the story. To truly gauge the health of your digestive motility, focus on the speed at which its contents travel. This is known as *Bowel Transit Time (BTT)*— the duration food takes from the moment it enters your digestive system to when it exits.

A well-functioning stomach processes its contents within 2-6 hours. Subsequently, the food moves through the small intestine for another 2-6 hours. Then, the colon takes over, processing it for an additional 10 to 15 hours. These times differ depending on factors such as diet, hydration, and physical activity. Thus, an optimal BTT ranges from 18 to 25 hours. This allows your body adequate time for digestion and nutrient absorption. It also prevents prolonged stagnation that can result in toxin build-up and microbial and fungal overgrowth.

Bowel Transit Time - Classical vs Modern view

8	16	25	48	72	hours

Bowel Transit Time

Classical View and the Lazy Gut Zone

Diarrhea   Normal   Lazy Gut   Constipation

Modern View (expanded "norm"):

Diarrhea   New Normal   Constipation

© 2022-2024 Anar R Guliyev, www.autoimmunityunlocked.org

Appendix 1: Figure 6.1 - Bowel Transit Time: the shift of definitions and the "Lazy Gut" concept

Unfortunately, many people nowadays surpass this optimal time-frame, often having a BTT of over 30 hours. It tends to be even higher among women, sometimes more than 40 hours, for reasons we'll discuss later. While this doesn't equate to constipation, many live with this gray zone condition—a state I refer to as "Lazy Gut." Chronic constipation is a known precursor for ulcerative colitis and colon cancer. While the "Lazy Gut" scenario is more subtle, it is also more widespread. It alters the microbiota and harms the gut lining, triggering chronic inflammation. Over time, this can lead to immune complications or even tumors. Because it often goes unchecked, its repercussions compound over years or even decades. Overlooking this issue is partly to blame for the surge in colorectal cancer rates. The current lifetime risk is already higher than 4% and is on an upward trajectory.

Alarmingly, Lazy Gut has become so common that medical benchmarks have shifted. Figure 6.1 compares classical and modern views of the ideal bowel transit time. The previously accepted norm for transit time was 15-25 hours. Any substantial deviations, especially consistent ones, were cause for concern. A BTT of 48 hours was labeled as constipation. Yet, contemporary guidelines only classify constipation as a BTT of more than 72 hours, with 30 to 40 hours now considered acceptable. This "new norm," once correctly considered weak motility, is what I refer to as "Lazy Gut."

If you have an autoimmune disease, you're likely also dealing with this condition.

Curious about your BTT? Testing is straightforward:

- Eat food that noticeably tints your stool, and record the ingestion time.
- Choose an easy marker, such as 4-6 g of *activated charcoal* for a black hue or 2-4 whole beets for a red tint.
- When you pass stool tinted with the color of the food, calculate the duration that has elapsed. That's your BTT.
- You may want to check it several times, as BTT varies widely depending on your food intake, hydration, and physical activity.

Your gut motility matters. Besides digestion, it is also crucial for microbiome, immune, liver, and overall health. In brief, it's time to understand and optimize your BTT. As we progress, remember that all DILL+ factors are interlocked, and you need to address them in parallel.

GUT MOTILITY AND OTHER DILL+ FACTORS

EFFECT ON THE MICROBIOME – RIVER VS SWAMPS

Imagine standing beside a swift mountain brook, watching the fresh clear water cascade down the slopes. Now, contrast this with the languid flow of a valley river or the stillness of a pond or swamp. The fast-moving mountain stream rarely has issues with bacterial pollution. On the other hand, stagnant water in ponds and marshes becomes a breeding ground for microbes.

Similarly, your intestines are a hotbed of nutrients for bacteria. Strong and consistent motility is essential to prevent bacterial overgrowth, especially in the small intestine. This active movement ensures bacteria don't linger in one place for too long, supporting proper microbiome *Distribution*.

Besides this, the microbiome *Composition* is also affected by gut motility. Fishing enthusiasts know that fast-moving streams usually have a greater diversity of aquatic life. Similarly, in the gut, contents moving at an optimal rate promote a more varied microbiota. A stagnant environment favors the overgrowth of certain aggressive bacteria in the upper segments of the intestine. As they occupy more niches, they rob the less dominant ones of resources and flood them with produced toxins. This effect spreads downstream and skews all ecosystem niches. Research confirms that those with a fast bowel transit time have a more diverse array of beneficial bacteria than those with longer transit times.

DILL+ Vicious Cycles: Lazy Gut

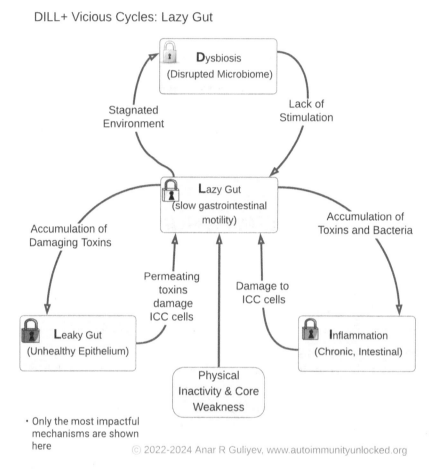

Appendix 1: Figure 6.2 - DILL+ Vicious Cycles: Lazy Gut (slow gastrointestinal motility)

This is why the so-called *low-FODMAP diet* can become a problem. Many turn to it in an attempt to control *SIBO (small intestinal bacterial overgrowth)*. In the short term, it reduces bacterial overgrowth and inflammation. However, the limitations on fiber and some other nutrients result in slower intestinal movements. This creates the perfect environment for unhealthy gut bacteria (and fungi) to flourish and undermines gut lining health. So, in the long run, it is like a suppressed underground movement biding its time for the perfect moment to stage a coup. Unlike the low-FODMAP diet, the 5R+ System targets the root of the problem, improving gut motility in parallel with other mechanisms that control bacterial growth.

The link between the microbiome and gut motility is a two-way street. Just as the movement of contents through the intestines is an important environmental factor for the microbiome, the microbiota impacts the passage of food through the digestive tract. Animal studies show that a lack of intestinal microbes results in impaired peristalsis. What's more, reintroducing these bacteria significantly improves gut activity. One reason for this is that beneficial gut bacteria produce several compounds essential for optimal gut motility. Therefore, in a state of good gut health, these two factors support each other. However, in disease, they create a vicious cycle. This is why we target all DILL+ factors at the same time. *Repopulating the Microbiome* helps to *Reawaken the Lazy Gut* and vice versa.

See also:
- Key 1 ➤ Microbiome Distribution.
- Key 1 ➤ Healthy Digestion to Fix Microbiota Distribution.

CHRONIC TOXIC LOAD

Every digestive process results in by-products, some being more harmful than others. For instance, when proteins decay, they produce particularly harmful toxins. This is one reason protein-rich foods place a heavier burden on both the immune and digestive systems.

Adding to that, the trillions of gut bacteria all excrete waste. As such, they don't necessarily make the gut cleaner. It can be even worse with an unhealthy microbiota, as in the case of SIBO. Simply put, you can't stop the waste production from chemical and microbial activities in your digestive system.

If left unchecked, this toxic waste will wreak havoc on the whole body. In the gut, it alters the environment of the microbiota, affecting its *Composition*. It also damages the gut epithelium, leading to complications such as *Leaky Gut* and other intestinal lining disorders. Furthermore, deeper penetrating toxins can harm other tissues within the digestive tract. These include the *Interstitial Cells of Cajal (ICC)*, further weakening gut motility. The result is a build-up of even more toxins—a vicious cycle, one of the many observed in the DILL+ factors.

> Interstitial cells of Cajal (ICCs) are specialized pacemaker cells located in the gastrointestinal tract (GIT), gallbladder, bile ducts, and urinary bladder. They generate impulses, which control the rhythm of muscle contractions in these organs. A deficiency of ICCs results in poor GIT muscle tone and contractions, making them essential for normal gut motility.

The damage doesn't remain localized. These toxic by-products can seep into your bloodstream, further burdening the liver and other organs. It can even impact the brain. Recent studies have highlighted the link between the microbiome and digestive health, and brain health. It is referred to as the *gut-brain axis*. It may be a newer area of medicine, but the concept isn't new. For a long time, people have associated "brain fog" with digestive issues and noted improved mental clarity during fasting.

Furthermore, many toxins can trigger immune reactions. The resulting chronic inflammation exhausts the immune system and causes it to malfunction.

A critical factor in all these issues is the slow movement of the contents through your gut. Healthy motility normally expels waste from the system quickly, preventing its prolonged effects. It is like the trash collection service that keeps your neighborhood streets clean, except it does not take days off.

See also:

- Key 1 ➤ Help Your Liver
- Consequences of Chronic Inflammation

LAZY GUT AND DIARRHEA

It might seem puzzling: How can a "lazy gut" lead to episodes of diarrhea? Surprisingly, this link is common, and understanding it is essential for your digestive health.

A lazy gut doesn't always mean *slow* but rather a *passive* progression of gut contents with little control from the bowel muscles. Sometimes, such passive flow becomes much faster than it should be. One reason for this is poor absorption. Excess water remains in the intestines when an unhealthy gut lining cannot efficiently absorb it. This makes the contents more liquid, abnormally speeding up the flow, which results in diarrhea. Additionally, certain toxins can irritate the intestine, causing it to dump food more rapidly. This is often caused by *dysbacteriosis* (a *disrupted microbiome*). For similar reasons, diarrhea occurs in many infectious gut diseases and food poisonings.

Note this is not a case of active "gut motility." Quite the contrary. The gut contents don't move due to active propulsion by peristalsis waves; rather, they flow passively, often without thorough digestion and absorption. This flow can be volatile, shifting rapidly between diarrhea and constipation. This is exactly what is experienced by many people with *IBS* or *Crohn's disease*. Picture a boat with a broken engine, its movements dictated more by external elements than the captain's hand, often remaining stationary or swaying with the whims of wind and currents.

 You need a reliable engine for your boat!

A well-functioning gut operates consistently, even if you skip meals for a day or two. Such stability sustains a healthy microbiome environment and effectively removes the toxins.

In summary, if you have sporadic diarrhea, it could be a sign of a lazy gut. Don't be tempted to skip the tactics outlined in this DILL+ section, including *prokinetic* foods. The 5R+ system aims to **normalize** gut movement, not just accelerate it. Of course, always consult with your doctor about your unique situation.

INFLAMMATION

You've likely noticed that when any part of your body, such as your joints, is inflamed or swollen, it becomes less active and more difficult to move. Inflammation alters the tissues, reducing their natural motion. This is true not only for external body parts; the intestine can be similarly affected. As previously discussed, people with autoimmune conditions usually have hidden chronic inflammation in their intestines. It often goes unnoticed due to the lack of explicit symptoms. Addressing this inflammation can enhance gut motility.

See also:

• Key 2 ➤ Inflammation: Reduce.

DAMAGE TO INTERSTITIAL CELLS OF CAJAL (ICC)

The greatest impact of intestinal inflammation on motility is the damage it causes to the Interstitial Cells of Cajal (ICC). Nestled within the gut wall, these cells are responsible for peristalsis, the rhythmic muscle movements that push food through the digestive tract. However, when the intestines are inflamed, ICC cells can be impaired, directly affecting intestinal muscle contractions.

Sometimes, problems begin with an acute gastrointestinal infection or food poisoning. Not only can these issues cause Leaky Gut and Dysbiosis, but the damage can go deeper, harming the ICC cells. For this reason, I recommend a brief spell of water fasting, followed by a *Green Basket* diet during and immediately after such conditions. This gives the gut time to recover.

More often, damage accumulates over time from the ongoing effects of toxins and constant low-level inflammation, typically due to an unhealthy microbiota or leaky gut. It is easy to see how detrimental processes reinforce each other, forming vicious cycles.

Interestingly, sugar is another frequent cause of damage to the ICC. I've lost count of the many reasons to cut sugar from your diet. In this case, studies have found that people with chronic high blood sugar have fewer ICC cells. This also means that if you are dealing with diabetes or pre-diabetes, it is essential to consult your doctor for effective blood sugar management.

Now for the good news. Unlike most other nerve cells, the enteric nervous system and ICC cells can regenerate! First, reduce inflammation, minimize toxic exposure, and normalize blood sugar levels. Then, allow time to work for you. Let's explore the main tactics you can apply to unlock this aspect of the DILL+ shackles.

See also:

• Bonus 3 ➢ Water-Fasting
• Appendix 1 ➢ Table 4.4

UNDERSTANDING THE ROOT CAUSE OF LAZY GUT

The root causes of passive gut motility include:

- Dysbiosis (see the *Key 1* section)
- Inflammation (see the *Key 2* section)
- ICC damage (often caused by *Inflammation*)
- Insufficient hydration
- Low core muscle tone
- Diet
- Psychological factors
- Prolonged use of *laxatives*
- Hypothyroidism (underactive *thyroid gland*)

Usually, it's a combination of several of these factors. In this section, we will explore each one. As always with the 5R+ System, I strongly recommend applying all tactics at the same time.

Note: *Hypothyroidism* (reduced *thyroid gland* function) falls outside this book's scope. If you believe you may have this condition, please consult your doctor.

WATER: DRINK RIGHT

The most frequent cause of slow bowel transit time is insufficient hydration.

Water is the only drink that fully meets your body's fluid requirements! Sadly, many people opt for various beverages instead—from juices or teas, in better scenarios, to harmful synthetic drinks. None of these alternatives can be your main source of hydration.

Yes, they are 99% water and contribute to your fluid intake. However, they also contain compounds that your body needs to metabolize and excrete, processes that themselves result in water loss. In other words, they give and take. It's akin to trying to wash something with tainted water. So, beverages do not offer the "free H_2O" your body needs for all life-sustaining activities, such as digestion, toxins removal, temperature control (through perspiration), and... healthy bowel function.

 Your body is almost two-thirds water, not other beverages.

The U.S. National Academies of Sciences recommends the following daily fluid intake:

- **Adult men:** 3.7 liters (about 15.5 cups).

- **Adult women:** 2.7 liters (roughly 11.5 cups).

About 20% of this intake comes from food and other drinks. That means the recommendation for drinking water is 3 liters for men and 2.1 liters for women. This is a baseline; factors like exercise, hot weather, breastfeeding, or certain medical conditions may necessitate more. The increased requirement can be covered only by water, not other drinks. Of course, a daily cup or two of juice, tea, or *ayran* (see *Bonus* 2) is fine, but it shouldn't cut into your pure water consumption.

Regularly consuming other beverages can lead to another kind of issue—an altered taste preference. Becoming accustomed to the taste of such drinks can make water less appealing, resulting in you hydrating less. It pays to consciously cultivate a preference for pure water over other drinks. Remember:

 Your palate is yours to control.

What is the best time to drink water? The timing of your water consumption is very important, as it can either aid or disrupt digestion. The ideal times include:

- **Before meals:** A significant amount of water is used during the digestive process. Therefore, it is important to consume enough water at least 15 minutes before eating to ensure its efficient absorption before digestion begins.
- **After digestion:** Refrain from drinking during or immediately after meals to avoid diluting digestive juices. Only start drinking after food is digested and has passed through the first part of the digestive tract. Depending on the food, wait between one to three hours after a meal. Light foods like fruits digest faster, whereas heavier foods like meat take longer.
- **Morning routine:** Jumpstart your gut every morning with 2-3 glasses of cool—not cold—water. Combined with physical activity, this activates healthy gut motility and ideally should

lead to bowel evacuation before breakfast. Make it a habit in order to maintain a healthy and clean intestine.

 Drink water before and between meals; not during or right after eating.

Here are a few important reminders:

- Avoid refrigerator-cold drinks; they are harmful to digestive health.
- Ensure your drinking water is free from harmful toxins, including chlorine and chloramine. Invest in a good water filtering system.
- Avoid regular consumption of distilled or reverse-osmosis water. If you use reverse-osmosis filtration, add a remineralization step.

Also see:
- Key 1 ➤ Don't Rush the Reactor
- Key 1 ➤ Stomach Acid ➤ Dilution of Digestive Juices
- Key 3 ➤ Obstacle #9: Chilled Food and Drinks
- Key 1 ➤ Chlorine and Related Compounds in Water

PHYSICAL ACTIVITIES FOR OPTIMAL BOWEL TRANSIT

A sedentary lifestyle is detrimental for numerous reasons, not least of which is its impact on gut motility. Being physically active is crucial for overall health, as well as many aspects of autoimmune disease. We will cover this in *Key 5*. Over and above general movement, certain exercises and muscle groups can specifically target the lazy gut condition. Let's explore how.

STRENGTHENING THE CORE AND ABDOMINAL MUSCLES

Strong abdominal and core muscles provide body stability. They also surround your internal organs, protecting them and ensuring their correct position. Furthermore, their consistent pressure is key for maintaining a toned gut with active motility.

There are two groups of muscles to consider:

- **Abdominal Muscles (Abs)**: Comprising four groups, these muscles form the front wall of your abdomen.
- **Core Muscles**: This broader group ensures 360-degree torso stability. It includes the abs and lower back, as well as the diaphragm and pelvic floor—the "ceiling" and "floor" of your midsection.

A weakened core and abs are often the cause of reduced gut motility, especially in women. However, exercises targeting these important muscle groups benefit everyone.

Key Exercises for strengthening the core and abdominal muscles are:

- **Crunches**: Primarily target the abs.
- **Planks**: Besides strengthening the abs, planks engage the broader core, spine-supporting muscles, and upper body. Plank modifications include side and reverse planks.

Mix crunches and planks in your routine for optimal results, focusing on all muscle areas. See the video guides in *Appendix 1*.

Safety First: Planks might be safer than crunches if you have a back injury or inflammation in the spine joints. Always consult with your doctor before starting a new exercise routine.

One last point: Since digestion requires considerable blood flow to the stomach and intestines, avoid exercise immediately after a meal. It takes at least an hour to digest fruits and up to five hours for protein-rich meals, especially meat. I suggest doubling this time as gut lining restoration may take longer in autoimmune conditions.

See also:
- Key 5 ➢ Physical Exercises
- Appendix 1 ➢ Videos 6.3, 6.4, 6.5

CHEWING

Remarkably, muscle activity in your mouth triggers corresponding actions in your gut. Thus, when you chew your food, it stimulates nerve reflexes that enhance gut motility. As such, thorough mastication (chewing) is one of the most underestimated aspects of a healthy lifestyle. It is so critical that it is highlighted in *Keys 1, 3,* and now, *Key 4* of our system.

See more:
- Key 1 ➢ Mastication and Salivation — The Underrated Duo
- Key 3 ➢ Obstacle #7: Insufficient Mastication

FLUSHING THE GUT: AYURVEDIC SHANKHA PRAKSHALANA TECHNIQUE SIMPLIFIED

Ayurveda, the traditional Indian medical system, has accumulated a vast array of health principles and practices over centuries of empirical observation. One such practice is *Shankha Prakshalana*, an intensive intestine cleansing technique that can be a valuable addition to your toolkit.

This method involves drinking salty water and performing certain poses and exercises to flush it through the digestive tract. What piqued my interest was the ingenious combination of exercises that stimulate gut peristalsis. While its primary goal is a thorough cleanse— confirmed when clear water exits the system—you often do not need its full intensity. We can adapt this technique to lesser objectives, such as promoting motility and aiding the movement of gut contents. This can be particularly beneficial to combat 'Lazy Gut' stagnation, a situation where the intestines are not active enough.

The simplified technique requires less water, reduces the exercise duration and the number of repetitions, and has several advantages for our purposes:

- It's quicker and easier to do.
- It's gentler on the intestinal ecosystem, allowing more frequent use. **Note**: The complete Shankha Prakshalana should not be done often.
- It is generally better tolerated and comes with fewer medical contraindications.

Warning: Shankha Prakshalana is not advised for pregnant or breastfeeding women or those with certain gastrointestinal disorders. Always consult your doctor before embarking on this or any other cleansing regimen.

How to Execute the Technique:

1. Ensure your stomach is empty. Refrain from eating at least

five hours before the procedure to prevent undigested food contaminating the lower gut sections.

2. Prepare salty water by mixing 1-2 tablespoons of salt into one liter of water. The salt ensures water remains in the gut by creating a high osmotic pressure, preventing absorption into the bloodstream. The exercises then guide this water volume through the entire digestive tract.

3. Drink 2-4 glasses of salty water. If you find the taste unpleasant, a splash of lemon juice can make it more palatable.

4. Complete 1-2 rounds of the recommended exercises, around 30 repetitions each. For a visual guide, refer to Video 6.6 in *Appendix 1*. Focus your attention on propelling water through the digestive tract rather than the external movements. Note: the hip movements begin on the right side because the colon progresses from right to left.

5. The goal is bowel evacuation within an hour. If needed, repeat the exercise sequence.

6. After this procedure, avoid heavy foods for the day, especially dairy, meat, and fish. Opt for lighter alternatives such as fruits or green salads and include prebiotic foods such as naturally fermented vegetables. Wait at least 2 hours after completing the exercise before eating.

This method is highly effective for gaining momentum with multiple DILL+ locks. Because it swiftly eliminates toxins and immune triggers from the digestive system, it is beneficial for the following:

- **Inflammation Reduction**: Combining this technique with one or two days of water-fasting can notably reduce inflammation in the intestine and throughout your body.
- **Effective for the 'Reset' Technique**: Shankha Prakshalana is particularly powerful when integrated into the *'Reset'* step of *ERR (Eliminate, Reintroduce, Reset)*.
- **Preparation for Repair**: You can use the technique to cleanse the gut and set the stage for a prolonged restoration course,

as described in *Key 3*. This can involve water fasting, followed by an *elemental* or *quasi-elemental diet*, and finally, a *Green Basket* diet. The objective is to "wash" the gut lining and reduce toxic stress long enough for repair.

- **Normalization of Microbiota Distribution**: This procedure displaces large quantities of bacteria in your digestive system, shifting them downstream. This can offer prompt relief for *SIBO (Small Intestinal Bacterial Overgrowth)*. To maintain this effect, however, you need to employ all strategies from *Key 1*.
- **Toxin Removal during Die-off Reaction**: I recommend the Shankha Prakshalana technique as a rapid-response tactic to eliminate toxins of the *SIBO die-off reaction*.

See also:
- Appendix 1 ➤ Video 6.6
- Key 2 ➤ Eliminate-Reintroduce-Reset Technique (ERR)
- Key 3 ➤ What If I Compromise My Diet? How to Reset
- Key 3 ➤ Water-Fasting
- Key 3 ➤ Quasi-Elemental Diet
- Bonus 3. Food Baskets: Foods Ranked by Their Impact on the Gut-Microbiome-Immune Ecosystem
- Key 1 ➤ Other Tactics for Fixing SIBO and Normalizing Microbiome Distribution ➤ Healthy Motility
- Key 1 ➤ Die-off Reactions

YOUR FOOD AND GUT MOTILITY

Your diet influences the rate at which food passes through your digestive tract. Some foods slow down the movement of gut contents, while others promote a more acceptable pace. In this chapter, we'll explore which food components you should avoid and those that support healthy gut motility, including:

- Fiber
- Prokinetics
- Oils
- Minerals

> Prokinetic foods stimulate the contraction of muscles in the stomach and intestines, thus promoting faster movement of food through the digestive system.

WHAT TO AVOID

 Often, eliminating bad elements paves the way for improvement more effectively than introducing good ones.

SUGAR

First on the list is our old, well-known offender: sugar. If the previous 5R+ tactics haven't motivated you to cut sugar from your diet, here's another compelling reason. Sugar disrupts gut activity in several ways:

- **Effect on ICCs:** High levels of sugar in the blood directly suppress the *interstitial cells of Cajal (ICC)*. The result is poor muscle tone and contractions.
- **Disrupted Microbiota:** Sugar wreaks havoc on the gut microbiome, promoting the growth of harmful bacteria and indirectly affecting motility.
- **Inflammation:** Earlier, we mentioned that sugar fuels inflammation in the digestive tract. This inflammation affects gut motility in two ways: first, as in any other part of the body, it hinders movement. Furthermore, it directly harms the ICC cells.
- **Stickiness:** Sugar can make the gut contents "sticky," which slows down its movement through the intestines.

 Cut out sugar to improve gut motility.

See also:
- Key 4 ➤ Gut Motility and Other DILL+ Factors
- Key 4 ➤ Inflammation ➤ Damage to Interstitial Cells of Cajal (ICC)
- Key 2 ➤ Inflammatory Foods

STARCH

In a similar vein, starch decelerates the bowel transit time. This is one reason I recommend cutting out starchy foods during the early stages of your healing journey and limiting them even after your gut has recovered.

 Do not let starch dominate your meals.

MEAT

Finally, meat-heavy meals also retard motility. You can moderate the impact by pairing meat with fiber-rich foods. This practice offsets several adverse effects of meat, allowing you to benefit from its protein content without impairing your motility and microbiota or creating a toxic load.

 Always combine meat with plenty of greens, herbs, and raw vegetables, including bitter ones.

THE FIBER PARADOX: WHY EAT WHAT YOU CAN'T DIGEST

Nutrient deficiencies are rare in most modern societies. The contemporary diet is generally high in carbohydrates, fats, and proteins. Even though it is often lacking in raw vegetables, the resulting low intake of vitamins and minerals is easily overcome with readily available supplements. However, a notable insufficiency exists in one vital component of the modern diet: *fiber*.

This fiber is mostly *cellulose*, a unique natural compound found in plants, closely related to starch. It is perhaps one of the most versatile substances, benefitting our lives in many ways: we build our houses with it (lumber), print our books on it (paper), cook over it (firewood), wear it (cotton and linen), and even eat it (veggies). Though we don't digest and absorb cellulose and other fiber as we do starch, it plays many roles within our digestive system:

- **Normalizes gut motility.** Fiber adds bulk to stool and stimulates intestinal contractions, facilitating smoother bowel movements.

- **Nourishes a healthy microbiome:** Fiber is a critical energy and nutrient source for beneficial gut bacteria.
- **SCFA production:** The bacterial fermentation of fiber results in *short-chain fatty acids (SCFA)*—an essential source of energy for the gut epithelium.
- **Acts as a filter:** Fiber absorbs toxins and helps remove them from your body. By keeping the gut environment cleaner, it prevents the toxic load from reaching your gut bacteria, blood, and internal organs.
- **Regulates cholesterol and sugar absorption:** By binding to cholesterol and slowing down the absorption of sugar, fiber is crucial for combating *type 2 diabetes* and *metabolic syndrome*.

Fiber has an immense impact on all DILL+ factors. This statement is backed by scientific research. The results of a clinical trial showed eating a high-fiber, plant-based diet led to the remission of *Rheumatoid Arthritis (RA)* in 41% of study participants. Yet, fiber deficiency in the contemporary diet is glaring. Proof of the lack of fiber is found in another study that compared the fiber content in people's stools. Alarmingly, those eating a modern Western diet had only 5 ounces of fiber in their stool compared to 16 ounces in people consuming a traditional African diet.

Addressing fiber deficiency is transformative, not only for *Lazy Gut* but also for the entire *microbiome ecosystem*.

 What you consume not only provides nutrients for your body but also shapes your microbiota's environment.

See also:
- Key 3 ➤ Nutrition For the Gut Epithelium

Two Types of Fiber: Tailoring Intake for Specific Conditions

There are two types of dietary fiber, each behaving differently within our digestive system:

- **Soluble fiber** dissolves in water, forming a gel-like substance in the gut.
- **Insoluble fiber** adds bulk to stool. It doesn't dissolve and remains largely unchanged as it travels through the digestive tract.

Both are crucial for optimal health and are provided naturally by a diverse whole plant-based diet. When your gut is healthy and your microbiome balanced, you can comfortably consume both types of fiber without worrying about their differences.

However, autoimmune diseases are often accompanied by varying degrees of *dysbiosis (disrupted microbiome)* and poor *intestinal lining* health. Under these circumstances, one or both types of fiber might worsen your problems, making it tempting to avoid fiber-rich foods altogether. While this may provide short-term relief, it is detrimental in the long run. Omitting fiber because of digestive discomfort is akin to shunning dumbbells due to weak muscles—it does not solve the root problem.

Instead, consider adjusting the balance between soluble and insoluble fibers as your condition demands. You can also apply the upcoming tips to help you tolerate them better. With such an approach, you can navigate this tricky territory while safely maximizing your fiber intake.

Meanwhile, continue following the 5R+ system, concurrently repopulating your microbiome (*Key 1*) and repairing your gut lining (*Key 3*). Both strategies will improve your fiber tolerance. The goal is to build strength and steadily transition to a diverse fiber-rich diet rather than sweeping the problems under the rug.

Warning: Consult your doctor to determine the most effective approach tailored to your specific condition.

See also:
- Appendix 1 ➤ Table 6.7

SOLUBLE FIBER

Soluble fiber is usually not a concern for people with *Leaky Gut* condition only. It is soft and unlikely to physically irritate sensitive intestines. However, its spongy nature means it is easily fermentable by bacteria, potentially worsening *Disrupted Microbiome* issues.

A high intake of soluble fiber, coupled with an overpopulation of bacteria in the upper intestine, can lead to excessive fermentation, gas, bloating, and cramps. Such an increase in fermentation is especially problematic for people affected by conditions such as *Small Intestinal Bacterial Overgrowth (SIBO)* or *Irritable Bowel Syndrome (IBS)*.

Here are a few tips on how to avoid these symptoms:

- **Better digestion**: Apply all tactics outlined in *Key 1* to boost digestive activity, including optimizing stomach acidity and bile production.
- **Meal Spacing and Water-Fasting.**
- **Suppress bacterial activity**: Add plenty of spices, herbs, and bitter vegetables to your meals. These can spoil the party for bacteria. They prevent excessive fermentation, thus helping to control bacteria populations.
- **Shift your dietary fiber intake to more *insoluble* fiber**: It is not easily fermentable by gut bacteria, making insoluble fiber a poor source of fuel and nutrients. Such a lack of food starves the bacteria in the upper gut. Insoluble fiber also counteracts SIBO by sweeping through the digestive tract, keeping the contents moving—acting as a broom for your intestines.

As you address the *Dysbiosis* DILL+ factor, you will become more tolerant of soluble fiber.

See also:

- Key 1 ➤ Healthy Digestion to Fix Microbiota Distribution
- Key 1 ➤ Healthy Digestion to Fix Microbiota Distribution ➤ Power of Herbs, Spices, and Other Foods to Control Microbial Growth

INSOLUBLE FIBER

Since insoluble fiber is not easily fermented by gut bacteria, it reduces the chances of gas, bloating, and other issues caused by a *Disrupted Microbiome Distribution*. Even though it is physically tougher, a healthy digestive system usually tolerates it well. However, it can be problematic if your gut lining is compromised. As a result, the roughness of insoluble fiber can aggravate irritation and damage in an already vulnerable gastrointestinal lining in conditions such as *Irritable Bowel Syndrome (IBS)*, *Inflammatory Bowel Disease (IBD)*, *Crohn's Disease*, and *Ulcerative Colitis*.

As highlighted in *Key 3*, overcoming severe gut epithelium conditions requires gentle and mechanically pre-processed food. Here are a few tips for those who don't tolerate insoluble fiber well:

- **Choose soft fiber sources**: Avoid foods containing very hard fiber (like cabbage, cauliflower, carrots, or celeriac). Instead, choose gentler options such as those from the *Green Basket*, including "soft" vegetables and leafy greens like dill, parsley, scallions, arugula, and baby spinach. Their softer, insoluble fiber is easier on your gut.
- **Add mechanical processing**: Use a food processor or blender to prepare green vegetable smoothies. Breaking down the insoluble fiber further reduces their abrasiveness. Instead of a hard scrubbing brush, you now have a gentle soft broom sweeping through your digestive system.
- **Chew thoroughly**: Not only does chewing grind and soften the fiber, it also releases saliva, which is essential for gut epithelium regeneration.
- **Shift your dietary fiber intake to more s*oluble* fiber.** It is fermented by beneficial gut bacteria to produce *Short Chain Fatty Acids (SCFA)*, essential for gut lining health.

 You want a soft broom, not a scrubbing brush.

Implement tactics from *Key 3* to speed up the *Repair* of your intestinal lining. As your gut heals, your fiber tolerance will improve, enabling the gradual introduction of more fiber-rich foods.

	Soluble Fiber	Insoluble Fiber
Types	• Pectin • Gums • Inulin • Glucans • Fructans	• Cellulose • Lignin • Hemicellulose
Properties	• Softer, gel-forming. • Fermentable by gut bacteria.	• Rough, insoluble. • Less fermentable by gut bacteria.
Can cause problems in people with	• Disrupted Microbiome Distribution	• Leaky Gut and unhealthy intestinal lining.
Mitigate issues by	• Bitter herbs, spices and other tactics to suppress bacterial activity. • See Key 1 section.	• Thorough mastication, opting for soft greens, and mechanical processing. • See Key 3 section.
Sources	• Fruits, berries—fresh and dried. • Vegetables: Carrots, Onions, Garlic, Leeks, Chicory, Dandelion, Jerusalem artichoke, Asparagus, Cucumbers, Zucchini, Squash, Avocado, Okra. • Kelp • Legumes/Pulses: Beans, Lentils, Peas • Chia seeds, Oats, Flaxseed • Psyllium (also acts as insoluble fiber, a bulk-forming laxative)	• Leafy Greens: Spinach, Arugula, Parsley, Kale, Swiss chard, celery. • Vegetables: Broccoli, Cauliflower, Brussels sprouts, Bok choy, Beets, Carrots, Turnips, Parsnips, Daikon, Radishes, Cucumbers, Zucchini, Squash, Avocado, Okra. • Legumes/Pulses: Beans, Lentils, Peas • Wheat bran • Psyllium (also acts as a source of soluble fiber)
Notes	• Potatoes, yams, and other starchy vegetables are high in starch and low in fiber. It is best to reduce or avoid them. • All plants contain both soluble and insoluble fiber, though the proportions vary. • Animal products contain zero fiber.	

Appendix 1: Table 6.7 - Two types of fiber: Tailoring your intake for specific conditions

Crohn's, IBD, **and** *Ulcerative Colitis* **Patients**: Be extra cautious when introducing tougher fibers, as they could worsen intestinal damage. Start with an elemental or quasi-elemental diet and gradually introduce *Green Basket* vegetables once you experience stable improvements. In the case of ulcers, this step takes longer than with other autoimmune conditions.

Note: Always consult with your doctor before making any changes to your diet.

See also:

• Key 3 ➢ Elemental and Semi-Elemental Diets

• Key 3 ➢ Quasi-Elemental Diet

• Key 3 ➢ Obstacle #7: Insufficient Mastication

• Bonus 3. Food Baskets: Foods Ranked by Their Impact on the Gut-Microbiome-Immune Ecosystem

PROKINETIC AND LAXATIVE FOODS

As previously discussed, fiber is essential for healthy gut motility. You can enhance its benefits with certain plant foods, categorized as natural *prokinetics* and natural *laxatives*. For our purposes, we will list them together. Incorporate the following into your diet as food products, not medications, and consume them in moderation:

• Ginger
• Artichoke (Globe artichoke)
• Peppermint
• Anise
• Fennel seeds, Caraway seeds
• Amla
• Figs
• Damsons, Prunes
• Olive and flaxseed oils
• Watermelon
• Naturally fermented vegetables

Dried fruits generally promote gut motility due to their high fiber content. However, figs, damsons, and prunes, as well as prune juice, are particularly effective. They contain a type of carbohydrate called *sorbitol* that acts as a *laxative*.

Olive and flaxseed oils also have mild laxative properties. They reduce inflammation, trigger the release of bile, and soften stools by acting as a lubricant. A few tablespoons of oil, taken on an empty stomach in the morning, can improve motility in many cases.

Traditionally made sauerkraut and other fermented vegetables help motility in several ways: they are fiber-rich, provide probiotic bacteria to support your microbiome, and their spicy ingredients and acid content stimulate all digestive functions.

Finally, *herbal bitters* have a prokinetic effect. However, they can have side effects and contraindications. I do not recommend using them without a specific need and a doctor's advice.

MAGNESIUM

A magnesium deficiency is another frequent cause of constipation. It also plays a role in other 5R+ strategies. For this reason, those with low magnesium levels can benefit from taking supplements. The recommended daily dose for adults is 400 mg for males and 300 mg for females.

BILE AND GUT MOTILITY

In addition to its crucial role in the microbiome, healthy bile production influences gut motility through certain bile acids that act as laxatives or *prokinetics*. Their modulating effect is complex, though. On the one hand, they delay gastric emptying and ensure better stomach digestion. On the other, they stimulate peristalsis in the small intestine, speeding up its transit time.

So, improving liver health and bile quality directly targets both the *Dysbiosis* and *Lazy Gut* locks of DILL+.

See also:
• Key 1 ➤ Bile and Liver Health

WATER-FASTING FOR ACTIVE MOTILITY

At first glance, it seems contradictory: how can abstaining from food speed up the movement of gut contents? The important keyword is WATER-fasting. Unlike religious fasting, it involves consuming generous amounts of water. This practice enhances gastrointestinal motility, helping in several ways:

- **Hormonal Stimulation:** Water-fasting activates certain hormones essential for healthy motility. This will be covered shortly.
- **Reducing Inflammation:** Giving your gut a break can reduce inflammation and help tissues heal, improving their movement.
- **Positively Impacting the Microbiome:** Water fasting reduces overgrowth in the upper part of the intestine and shifts it to the lower segment, thus correcting *microbiome distribution*. It also improves the *microbiome composition* as certain beneficial bacteria, like *Akkermansia*, thrive in periods of hunger.

It might seem bizarre: Why is there still "output" if I'm not eating? Indeed, this question underscores the complexity of your digestive system. While it is best known for the digestion of food and absorption of nutrients, it is also instrumental in removing toxins from the blood, and thus, from the entire body. Also, your gut is teeming with billions of bacteria, many perishing daily. Up to 30% of stool is bacteria—dead or living. Adding to the tally of dead material in your gut are the dying cells of your intestinal lining—recall their rapid life cycle.

All these processes continuously produce waste, so there is always trash to expel, even without food intake. Interestingly, when a person's gut and microbiome are both healthy, a 1-2 day water fast doesn't interrupt the regularity of gut evacuation. It typically remains at once or twice a day. Given this, one wonders how some people can eat more frequently than waste is expelled.

 If the output cannot match the input, it spells trouble for any transit system.

See also:
- Key 3 ➤ Water-Fasting
- Key 1 ➤ Other Tactics for Fixing SIBO and Normalizing Microbiome Distribution ➤ Meal Spacing and Water-Fasting

HUNGER HORMONES

As previously noted, a moderate sense of hunger is not only harmless but also essential for several body functions. One of its key roles is regulating gastrointestinal motility.

When your stomach and upper intestines are empty, "hunger" hormones, *ghrelin* and *motilin,* are produced. As well as making you feel hungry and stimulating your appetite, they also activate peristalsis, ensuring efficient waste removal. This happens when your stomach "growls," and you feel empty and mildly uncomfortable. Such a boost in appetite hormones is one of the reasons a day of fasting can significantly improve gut motility.

Today's pervasive snacking culture means people seldom experience extended periods of having an "empty stomach." Constant grazing inhibits the production of hunger hormones, depriving the digestive system of its natural rhythm. Indeed, continuous snacking throughout the day is known to cause constipation.

So, the next time hunger strikes, remember its broader benefits. It's not only about feeding the body; it's also about keeping it running smoothly.

See also:

• Key 3 ➢ Obstacle #8: Snacking and Frequent Meals

PSYCHOLOGICAL FACTORS

Did you know that psychological factors also play a role in slowing down gut motility? Often, this is due to unhealthy habits like ignoring the need "to go." Here are some ideas based on cognitive behavioral therapy that you can use to improve the frequency of your bowel movements:

- **Heed the Signal:** Don't procrastinate when your body gives you the cue that you need to make a trip to the bathroom. Delaying bowel movements because you're too busy or it's an inconvenient time interrupts the gut's natural rhythm.
- **Mental Setup:** Consciously encourage active motility. Set a mental goal to evacuate your bowels more than once a day. This might sound odd because the gut muscles operate on autopilot, unlike the easily controlled skeletal muscles in your limbs. However, your mindset can influence their "program" and activity level.
- **Evening Routine:** Establish a cleansing ritual before bedtime, allowing your gut to rest at night without the burden of toxins. Initially, your good intentions may seem ineffective. However, with consistent practice and the addition of physical activity, your gut can synchronize with your brain. In the beginning, a cup of ginger tea or prune

juice may help stimulate a pre-bedtime bowel movement, but this nudge will become unnecessary over time.

- **Morning Routine:** Similarly, begin your morning by clearing your gut. Before breakfast, drink a generous amount of cool water, followed by physical exercise. This practice not only enhances gut health but also instills vigor for the day ahead.
- **Physical Exercise is Key:** Schedule exercises that target core and abdominal muscles into your evening and morning routines to promote efficient gut motility.

See also:
- Key 4 ➤ Strengthening the Core and Abdominal Muscles

CAREFUL WITH LAXATIVES

Unfortunately, many people hold the view that health solutions come in the form of a pill. In the healthcare system, patients are often seen as "customers," and since we are told "the customer is always right," such pills will always be sold. It is a classic case of supply and demand. Instead of treating the cause of the problem, though, this approach offers only symptomatic relief. It ignores your body's overall health and long-term well-being.

Constipation is no exception. *Laxative* medications are widely available and commonly used, even though their prolonged use is destructive. Unfortunately, many "customers" are still content to cut corners, and the allure of a quick fix persists. Some people even develop a dependence on such medication, becoming "laxative addicts." Although the strategies for gut health covered in this book demand significant effort and fundamental changes to your lifestyle, they pave the way for a genuine holistic solution.

On a side note, I am intrigued by the number of people abusing laxatives in their quest to lose weight. There's a persistent search for a magic potion, a belief that adding something to the diet can help shed pounds. Pure logic suggests it is not about "what else to eat" but "what to remove." Misusing laxatives is often seen as an alternative to smaller portions as it interrupts normal digestion and absorption of energy and nutrients. You eat, but you don't eat—your food is expelled. Yes, it reduces calorie intake, but it opens the door for a host of other problems.

 Nature cannot be tricked. The fine for trying is often paid in the currency of health.

The importance of a thorough, uninterrupted digestion process has been extensively covered. Remember, it's not just about calories. It shapes the ecosystem of your microbiome and immune cells, affecting your overall health. Apart from this, an imbalanced microbiome is also a significant contributor to obesity, along with a flawed diet. The nutritional guidance laid out in this book naturally leads to weight normalization by addressing them both.

 You do not need to deceive nature when you can collaborate.

Let's get back to laxative medications. The regular use of laxatives often diminishes gut motility and, ironically, can cause *constipation*. When overstimulated, an organ becomes dependent on that stimulus and, over time, builds a resistance to it. This desensitization is akin to endlessly whipping a horse: it eventually becomes unresponsive to gentler prods and requires more and more force to comply. Not to mention, its health deteriorates. If you are habitually using laxatives, even as infrequently as once a week, it's time to stop. Seek medical advice, reassess your approach, and consider the lifestyle changes we've discussed.

Most laxatives, even those available over the counter (OTC), are intended for sporadic or short-term use. They are useful tools for specific purposes like initiating gut cleansing, purging *SIBO Die-off*, resetting dietary missteps, or briefly addressing spikes in inflammation. However, even in these situations, physical exercises might be a more natural choice.

The only laxative category deemed safe for long-term use is *bulk-forming* agents. They are fiber supplements, similar to dietary fiber. You can improve their effectiveness by combining them with a softener, like olive oil. If you must turn to other OTC laxatives for a single occasion, opt for conservative varieties, like the *osmotic* category—*magnesium salts, Milk of Magnesia, Lactulose,* or *polyethylene glycol (PEG).* Of course, the cardinal rule always stands: Get advice from your doctor before making any decisions about medications or supplements.

Our goal in *Key 4* is to *Reawaken* natural gastrointestinal motility and eliminate the need for pharmaceuticals.

See also:

- Key 1 ➤ Die-off Reactions
- Key 2 ➤ Eliminate-Reintroduce-Reset Technique (ERR) ➤ How to Reset Faster
- Key 3 ➤ What If I Compromise My Diet? How to Reset
- Key 4 ➤ Flushing the Gut: Ayurvedic Shankha Prakshalana Technique Simplified
- Key 4 ➤ The Fiber Paradox: Why Eat What You Can't Digest

✔ PRACTICAL RECAP

DILL+ Lock: **L**azy gut.
5R+ Key Strategy: **R**eawaken Healthy Gut Motility.

Below are concise highlights of actionable steps for Key 4. For detailed information, please refer to the relevant chapters in this section.

- **Hydration:**
  - Baseline water recommendations:
    - Men: 3 liters.
    - Women: 2.1 liters.
  - Other drinks should not cut into your pure water consumption.
  - Avoid drinking during or immediately after meals.
- **Exercise and Physical Activity:**
  - Strengthen the core and abdominal muscles:
    - Crunches.
    - Planks.
  - Simplified Ayurvedic Shankha Prakshalana technique.
- **Diet and Nutrition:**
  - Avoid sugar.
  - Do not let starch dominate your meals.

- Avoid excessive meat. Combine it with plenty of greens, herbs, and various raw vegetables, including bitter ones.
- Thorough chewing.
- Increase fiber intake:
  - Soluble.
    - To prevent issues: suppress bacterial activity.
      - Spices, herbs.
      - Bitter vegetables.
      - Improve digestion.
      - Meal spacing and water-fasting.
  - Insoluble.
    - To prevent issues: You want a soft broom, not a scrubbing brush.
      - Choose softer fiber sources.
      - Add mechanical processing.
      - Chew well.
- Magnesium.
- Prokinetic foods
- Laxative foods, oils, stool softeners.
- **Routine and Lifestyle:**
  - Water-fasting.
  - Psychological factors for active motility.
    - Evening routine.
    - Morning routine.
  - Avoid laxative abuse.

KEY 5. FACTORS BEYOND DIGESTIVE HEALTH: RECONDITION

In our quest to combat autoimmune diseases, we've focused on three interrelated pillars: the microbiome, the intestinal immune system, and the digestive tract. It makes sense, given that these domains make up your body's ecosystem, where most immune cells reside and evolve.

Four of the 5 "R" strategies and DILL+ locks are directly related to digestive health and the microbiome:

- Repopulate the Disrupted Microbiome
- Reduce Inflammation
- Repair the Leaky Gut
- Reawaken the Lazy Gut.

This final section introduces the fifth "R"—Reconditioning Factors Beyond Digestive Health. It broadens our approach, exploring other factors affecting the immune system and the tactics you can employ to overcome them.

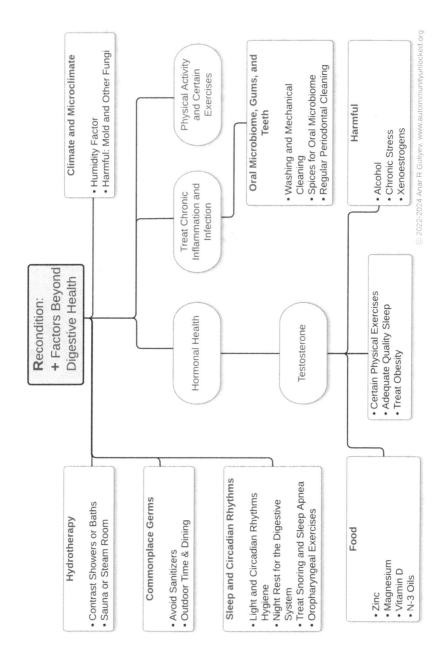

Appendix 1: Figure 7.0.1 - Key 5 Tactics. Recondition Factors Beyond Digestive Health.

THE HYGIENE PARADOX: WHEN CLEANING BACKFIRES

HYGIENE HYPOTHESIS AND "OLD FRIENDS" EFFECT

In 1989, British physician David Strachan made an intriguing observation: a link between increased hygiene during childhood and the onset of allergies later in life. From these insights, he proposed the *"Hygiene Hypothesis,"* believing the underlying mechanism could be an imbalance in T-lymphocyte counts. Time has shown this explanation to be too simplistic, though not wrong. Mounting evidence suggests that the cleaner your surroundings and the fewer bacterial interactions you have, the more likely you are to develop allergies and autoimmune diseases.

> Lymphocytes are a type of white blood cell, a large family of immune cells with two main classes: T-lymphocytes control your body's immune response and directly attack and kill infected and tumor cells. B-lymphocytes produce antibodies—proteins that target viruses, bacteria, and toxins.

It is well-established that exposure to a variety of microbes is essential for developing the immune system. Commonly referred to as the *"Old Friends"* hypothesis, it's also known as the *"Microbiome Depletion*

Hypothesis" or the "*Microbial Diversity Hypothesis.*" These names pinpoint the core issue:

 Low diversity in the skin microbiome undermines immune health.

The underlying mechanisms of this effect are complex and still not well understood. However, the *hormesis* principle offers some valuable insights. When your body is moderately challenged, it adapts, learning to function under various conditions. For instance, the brain needs challenges to remain sharp, muscles require physical activity to stay strong, and the heart benefits from regular cardiovascular exercises. Similarly, the immune system requires interaction with its natural enemies to learn how to function properly.

The key to immune system hormesis is the type and amount of stimulation, as well as sufficient recovery time. Of course, you want to avoid aggressive, dangerous pathogens. However, exposure to a range of milder bacteria engages and "trains" your immune cells without posing significant threats. While the gut microbiota takes center stage, microorganisms are not limited to the intestines. Rather, they are wide-spread throughout your body, occurring naturally on your skin, in your nose and mouth, and almost everywhere. We have more bacteria in our bodies than our own cells, and this population shapes our health in many ways.

Recent evidence supporting this theory emerged from a study comparing Karelian and Finnish populations. These two neighboring regions in Northern Europe share similar climates, genetics, and tradi-tions. However, due to socio-economic differences, Finns are exposed to less dust and common pathogens. The results of the study showed that they have a more than six-fold increase in allergy rates compared to their Karelian neighbors just across the river, who live in "less ster-ile" settings.

But don't dismiss hygiene entirely. You need to maintain a level of cleanliness that prevents dangerous infections from highly aggressive pathogens like those causing *hepatitis*, *tuberculosis*, and other diseases.

On the flip side, there are countless *"common germs"*—low-risk, mild bacteria—essential for your immune cells' fitness.

> Practice *targeted hygiene*—avoid hazardous pathogens and increase exposure to a diversity of mild *common germs*.

Most research emphasizes childhood as a critical period for immune system formation. Even so, the rotation and maturation of immune cells continue throughout life, making these effects relevant for adults, too, especially over extended periods.

See also:

• Key 2 ➤ Intermittent Hormesis

THE POWER OF BACTERIA TO MODULATE THE IMMUNE SYSTEM

Many years ago, a cycling accident taught me about the powerful influence of common bacteria on the immune system's behavior. During a dusk bike ride with my eldest son, I rode through some shrubbery. Later, I noticed the branches had scraped my skin, resulting in a soil-laden wound on my foot. By morning, severe inflammation had taken root, persisting for days. My usual approach for minor, less-contaminated scratches is baking soda compresses and iodine. This time, though, it fell short. Days later, faced with a purulent wound and a foot swollen beyond recognition, I reluctantly had to turn to stronger medical interventions.

However, I made an unexpected observation from this ordeal. Throughout the duration of the foot infection, my chronic joint inflammation—a signature symptom of my Rheumatoid Arthritis (RA)—seemingly disappeared. It was as though the infection had toggled a mysterious switch, neutralizing my RA more effectively than any prescribed medication. I realized what had happened. Pharmaceutical companies are on the hunt for effective *immunomodulators*—drugs that can change the immune system's structure and function—to treat autoimmune diseases.

Some bacteria are potent natural immunomodulators.

When immune cells confront a wide range of genuine threats, they optimize their function, ceasing misdirected attacks on the body's own tissues. Even brief encounters with common bacteria can stimulate the regulatory activity of specific T-lymphocytes, alleviating autoimmune conditions.

More extensive research in the field is necessary to identify the strains that yield the best effects. Seemingly, my biking mishap introduced me to some of them. Now, I don't recommend deliberately wandering barefoot through thorny bushes! Safer avenues exist, thanks to your skin's unique role in immune function.

SKIN MICROBIOME AND T-LYMPHOCYTES

Earlier, I mentioned the *hygiene hypothesis,* a theory linking an overly sanitized environment to abnormal *T-lymphocyte* counts. It is a key consideration in autoimmune disease because certain T-lymphocytes regulate immune responses, including the suppression of abnormal reactions.

> Antigen: A substance that triggers an immune response. Antigens include germs such as bacteria or viruses and environmental substances like food, pollen, or dirt.

Interestingly, an important stage of T-lymphocyte maturation occurs in the skin. In fact, at any given moment, over 20 billion of these cells pass through your body's outer surface—more than in your bloodstream. They come dangerously close to the "wild outside"—the broad range of germs and environmental dirt particles that frequent your skin. This continuous rotation of lymphocytes and antigens makes your skin the perfect training ground for immune cells.

The natural state for humans, which our ancestors thrived in for millennia, involves regular skin contact with "common dirt" and a variety of bacteria.

MORE TIME AND MEALS OUTDOORS

As previously mentioned, the key lies in exposure to a broad spectrum of **mild** agents and avoiding those that are overly harmful. This means engaging with *common dirt*—ideally in the form of organic soil and plants. The best way to do so is to venture outdoors in areas with an abundance of diverse vegetation. Activities such as *organic gardening*, hiking along nature trails, and camping outdoors are perfect examples of such exposure. Remember, the goal is to nurture a wide *variety* of microbiota.

 Add gardening to your list of hobbies.

Even your backyard provides a healthier environment than the inside of your house. Indoor dust, especially in urban settings, has a detrimental effect on your immune health. It's a cocktail of dead skin cells, dust mites, human hair, microplastics, and fabric fibers. With such a limited spectrum, dominated by synthetic materials and human antigens, it is the enemy of your immune system. Similarly, the clique of germs living on your furniture and within your rooms pales in comparison to the bacterial communities of fields and woods. Indoor spaces suffer from a lack of microbial diversity and an overgrowth of certain species, like harmful molds.

Make it a habit to open windows whenever you are inside. Letting in fresh air and direct sunlight fosters a healthier indoor microclimate, leading to a better bacterial ecosystem that ultimately influences your microbiome. In almost all cases, open windows create a much healthier environment than air conditioners.

Open windows are the absolute minimum you can do. Stepping out into your backyard is good, visiting the park is better, and camping in the forest is best. The more time you spend outdoors and the wilder the environment, the greater your antigen exposure, providing considerable benefits for your immune system.

Be that as it may, you don't need to be covered in mud like a medieval peasant from dawn to dawn. All it takes is an hour or two of regular contact with soil and vegetation. Even when you wash up later, the brief engagement with "weak enemies" has an *immunomodulatory* effect—adjusting (modulating) the behavior of your immune cells. Over time, an outdoor lifestyle can help cultivate a healthy micro-biome, inside and out.

There's a good chance you will ingest a minuscule amount of dirt. It's a good thing. As a matter of fact, I recommend dining outdoors whenever you can. The local germs find their way into your system, further enriching your microbiome. After all, this is the way humans have lived for millennia.

 Step outside and embrace a little dirt.

See also:
• Key 5 ➤ Microclimate: Small Changes Without a Big Move

NON-ORGANIC AGRICULTURE

In the previous section, you may have noticed that I deliberately emphasized *organic* gardening. It's not merely a buzzword; I hope it caught your attention. The reason is that non-organic fertilizers and pesticides are used to boost plant growth and control pests, but they also alter the soil's microbial population. So, when you work closely with the soil, your microbiome can be affected, too.

Every time you dig into the ground, tiny particles end up on your hands and face, and inevitably, some are swallowed. As with chemical food additives, safety regulations only consider the direct toxic effects of these chemicals on human bodies. They ignore the *selective pressure* they exert on your microbiome, altering it and thus affecting your immune system.

Studies suggest that farmers working with pesticides face an increased risk of *rheumatoid arthritis*. This is due to the direct chemical impact on the human body, as well as the indirect effects via micro-biota changes. So, immerse yourself in good old-fashioned gardening. Engage with healthy organic soil, and steer clear of pesticides and other harmful chemicals.

SANITIZERMANIA

While only a small number of people work with agricultural pesticides, many compromise their skin's healthy microbiome in other ways. One of the biggest modern-day problems is the widespread use of sanitizers, which skyrocketed during the COVID-19 pandemic. Are you aware of the health implications of using these products on your hands and in your home?

It's a common misconception that sanitizers safeguard you by eliminating only harmful germs. Unfortunately, they don't discriminate, and the milder, benign strains take the biggest hit. Consequently, aggressive and resistant germs flourish in the absence of competition. Dreaded *hospital infections* and "superbugs" are the result of the same mechanism. They are a problem in medical facilities where a relentless barrage of disinfectants and antibiotics paves the way for them by suppressing weaker bacteria.

Remember the lawn analogy from our discussion about gut microbiota? Just as a thriving cover of healthy grass naturally deters weeds, a robust skin microbiome safeguards the body. Beneficial bacteria occupy important *ecological niches*, making it hard for strangers to find space to settle. Disrupt this natural balance in the gut, skin, or any other organ, and you inadvertently create a void—an opportunity for aggressive invaders to take hold.

 You cannot just kill bacteria and have sterile skin unless you're in outer space. Fortunately, you do not need to.

The advice is simple. Ditch the sanitizers! Trust in the cleansing power of water, relied upon by many generations. Furthermore, to protect your skin's essential bacterial community, use regular soap when you need it—avoid "antibacterial" labels.

 Your skin needs its natural microbial population.

VEGETABLES: TO WASH OR NOT TO WASH?

Before we continue, let's address a potential misconception about the enrichment of your microbiome. It may seem like a good idea to eat unwashed vegetables. After all, it ensures the introduction of beneficial bacteria directly into your system. Be cautious! This approach is generally not recommended. Here's why:

- **Toxic Chemical Residue**: Modern agricultural practices rely on chemicals. Fruits and vegetables are often coated in harmful pesticides and other toxins.
- **Dangerous Germs and Parasites**: Unwashed vegetables can carry harmful infections like *Salmonella*, *Listeria*, and parasitic worms. Organic vegetables are not immune to this problem as manure is used to fertilize the crops.

 Our goal is exposure to a variety of mild common bacteria, not severe pathogens.

Vegetables that grow in, on, or near the ground are often the most contaminated. The soil can be riddled with animal feces, parasites, and other harmful agents. Eating these vegetables without proper washing exposes your body to these hazards in quantities that can overwhelm your immune system. On the other hand, fruits picked directly from trees are usually safer, provided they haven't been subjected to harmful chemical sprays or bird droppings. Use your judgment in this case.

Remember, a robust and diverse gut microbiota, along with healthy stomach acidity and bile production, equips your system to fend off many foodborne infections.

A special note on bat feces: Bats are reservoirs for a wide array of deadly viruses, many still being researched. Steer clear if you suspect any potential contamination from bats.

See also:

- Key 1 ➤ Overcoming Microbiota Inertia: Conquest or Immigration
- Key 1 ➤ Stomach Acid

ENVIRONMENT AND CLIMATE: WHERE YOU LIVE MATTERS

Throughout history, it has been observed that cold, damp conditions often worsen rheumatic ailments, especially arthritis. Even so, the other extreme isn't any better. Prolonged exposure to intense sunlight and heat can negatively impact many autoimmune diseases. Clearly, the connection between climate, environment, and disease is multifaceted and doesn't follow one simple rule. However, some climates are healthier than others for certain conditions.

I know several people who developed *Rheumatoid Arthritis (RA)* within a year of moving from the Mediterranean coast to the American Midwest or Canada. While their nutrition and lifestyle remained largely unchanged, a drastic climate shift appeared to be the primary trigger. In another compelling case, a woman's joint inflammation toggled on and off following her moves from one side of a mountain to the other. The problem was in the gorge on the north side. The almost perpetual shade of the mountain created a cool and humid environment, markedly different from the sunlit southern slope.

It's more than just the weather at play, though. A mere change in your surroundings can be a game-changer for your health. Sometimes, the problem is only in a specific house or office.

Undeniably, the environment and climate have a direct impact on bodily tissues. However, the link between these factors and immune health becomes clearer when we consider their influence on the microbiome. This chapter covers general trends and guidelines on climate, microclimate, and environment. We will also explore the changes you can make without having to move to a different geographic location.

THE EFFECT ON MICROBIOTA

Unlike an astronaut's space suit, your skin doesn't completely isolate you from your environment. On a microbial level, the boundary between the world outside your body and your internal ecosystem is blurred. Microorganisms migrate and interact; to them, you are merely a part of the landscape.

 Your body's microbiome is an extension of the microbial population of your surroundings.

As a result, environmental changes, including climate shifts, that affect the microbial population in your location, will also impact your inner microbiota. Thus, these external factors affect your immune cells, influencing disease activity. We know that certain symptoms, such as joint pain, intensify with approaching inclement weather. Similar microbial-driven changes are widespread in nature. A common example is *petrichor*, the distinct, earthy aroma accompanying rain. This scent comes from chemicals released by soil bacteria in wet weather. Additionally, the rapid growth of mushrooms following rainfall illustrates the quick response of fungi. A more infamous example is the mold growth that occurs in basements or attics when there's a leak —an issue so destructive that many insurance policies specifically exclude it.

Such microbial shifts in our environment are a threat not only to framing and drywall but also to flesh and blood. As highlighted in *Key 1*, fungal growth significantly endangers your microbiome and overall immune health. Molds and yeasts are often linked to immune system disorders, especially when they settle in your gut. Hence, unsurprisingly, the most harmful climatic conditions for people are those favoring fungal growth—damp places with limited sunlight.

CLIMATE: GOOD VS. BAD

Here are the main guidelines:

- Dry is better than humid.
- Warm weather is better than cold.
- Moderately sunny is better than shady.
- Higher elevations are better than lower ground.
- Good ventilation is better than stagnant air.

 Avoid damp, fungi-friendly places.

Important: Moderately warm and sunny conditions are ideal. Excessive sunlight can worsen some autoimmune conditions. Limit your direct sun exposure if you experience skin or eye inflammation.

MICROCLIMATE: SMALL CHANGES WITHOUT A BIG MOVE

Around 900 A.D., the great scientist and physician Muhammad ibn Zakariyya al-Razi was searching for the ideal location for a new hospital in Baghdad. In his quest to promote health and healing, he devised an ingenious method to identify the best spot. He placed pieces of meat inside wooden columns throughout the city, observed them for a few days, and chose the location where decomposition was slowest. He concluded that this area offered the healthiest microclimate, making it best for patient recovery.

This story illustrates how variations in landscape, soil type, elevation, and wind direction can yield significant differences. The effects on grass and trees are obvious. Even within the same backyard, you may notice that certain spots are preferred by different vegetation. Less obvious is the impact these factors have on the invisible microbial world. Furthermore, prolonged exposure to these environments can influence your personal microbiome.

Two homes in the same block, or even neighboring rooms in a building, can present different mold risks and germ populations.

Enhancing your surroundings doesn't always mean moving to an entirely new area.

Seek Sun, Elevation, and Ventilation

Avoid perpetually shady places. Rather, choose south-facing locations, be it the slope of a hill or the side of a large building. The opposite is true for those in the southern hemisphere—lean towards the northern side. These areas receive more sunlight, typically making them warmer and drier.

Elevation matters, too. Simply ascending 20-30 meters on a hill or selecting a higher floor in a tall building can mean a healthier microclimate—purer air, less humidity, and enhanced sunlight.

Keep a Tab on Humidity

Damp and mold go hand in hand. Fungi thrive when relative humidity is 80% or higher, especially in places rich in organic matter. Environments with a relative humidity of 40-50% are best for health and comfort.

Sick House

Even if you live in an area known for its healthy climate, your home or office might be undermining your well-being. This phenomenon isn't new; it's often termed "*sick house*" or "*sick building syndrome (SBS).*"

Research by the World Health Organization (WHO) in 2009 suggests that up to 50% of indoor environments in regions such as Europe, North America, Australia, India, and Japan grapple with significant mold problems. The prevalence is even higher in locales like river valleys and coastal areas.

Several factors contribute to this unhealthy indoor setting:

- Excessive humidity due to poor design, water damage, or both.

- Inadequate ventilation.
- Insufficient sunlight exposure.
- Contaminated air conditioning ducts.

How can you find the problem? Here's how to check:

- Professional air sampling and analysis is the gold standard for detection, though it can be costly.
- Do-It-Yourself mold test kits, available at many home improvement stores, are more affordable but less accurate.
- Check for common signs of a 'sick house':
  - Water condensation on windows or other surfaces.
  - Visible mold growth, especially the menacing black mold.
  - A noticeable moldy odor.
  - Badly maintained air conditioning systems with old or dirty ventilation ducts.
  - A history of water damage or known leaks. Look for dampness in the basement, dripping or rusty plumbing, or roof faults.
  - Homes built into hillsides or those perpetually shaded by the surrounding landscape.
  - Older homes tend to have such problems more often.

In extreme situations, relocating might be the best choice. However, often, a few targeted repairs can make a world of difference. Remember, molds thrive in the presence of moisture, oxygen, and organic matter. While mold spores are everywhere, altering the environment can make it inhospitable for fungi, improving the microbial population in your home. Here's what you can do:

Tackle humidity:

- Address all leaks without delay: Repair roofing, plumbing, and siding.
- Invest in a quality *dehumidifier*: Target a humidity level between 40-50%.

- Address problem areas: Basements are humidity magnets as moist air is heavier and moves down. Also, pay attention to the attic—check for and repair any minor leaks.
- If necessary, install a sump pump.
- Ensure good ventilation and sunlight penetration.

Remove decaying and mold-infested materials:

- Treat or replace moldy materials such as drywall, insulation, framing, masonry, or carpeting.
- Carpets trap dirt and moisture, making them a breeding ground for mold and other pathogenic germs. Rather, opt for hard flooring, which is easier to maintain.

Enhance Ventilation:

- Install fans: Use them consistently, particularly in damp-prone areas like bathrooms, kitchens, and laundry rooms.
- Windows are your friends: Keep them open as much as possible to refresh the indoor air.
- Open windows on opposite sides of the building and across different floors to promote steady airflow, which is essential for a healthy microclimate.
- To enhance this effect, strategically place fans to direct air outward through the windows.
- Weather conditions often make it impractical to keep your windows open all day. In such cases, identify the best time to ventilate: early mornings for hot climates and afternoons for cold ones.

Invite sunlight in:

- Open your curtains or blinds to prevent rooms from being continuously shaded.

Air Conditioning Systems and Vents

Pay special attention to all air conditioning and ventilation systems. When neglected, they quickly become breeding grounds for pathogens. Of particular concern is an old A/C or a unit in a building with a history of water damage or mold infestation. In such cases, professional cleaning is necessary. You may need to replace some parts of or even the entire A/C system.

It goes without saying that you should change A/C filters frequently, especially after high humidity or dirty construction and home repairs. Also, don't forget to clean all A/C vents and ducts regularly. For a thorough cleaning, consider a professional duct service. It's generally recommended every three years, but do it more often if there's a contamination risk.

In cold climates, your A/C may include a *humidifier* function. Due to its warm, damp environment, this part becomes a mold magnet. Clean it thoroughly and replace the humidifier pad and pipe regularly.

 The A/C system is your home's microbial "Achilles heel."

If your residence or office is in a large building, the situation becomes even more challenging. Even if your unit is clean, shared HVAC systems can spread germs from one area to another through the ventilation ducts. Regular mold tests can help identify these risks.

Finally, even with these precautions, limit A/C use.

Open windows and natural ventilation are almost always healthier options.

HORMONES. WHY DO FEMALES EXPERIENCE MORE AUTOIMMUNE CONDITIONS?

More than 85% of patients diagnosed with multiple autoimmune diseases are female. The reasons for this disparity include:

- Genetics
- Hormones
- Weaker stomach muscles, contributing to the "Lazy Gut" DILL+ factor.

This chapter focuses on the hormonal factors contributing to autoimmune diseases. First and foremost, females generally have higher levels of the hormone *estrogen*, which is known to stimulate the immune system. As such, elevated estrogen levels can increase the risk of abnormal immune reactions, including autoimmune responses. This is particularly clear when estrogen levels rise unnaturally.

On the flip side, *testosterone*, a hormone predominantly higher in males, has an immunosuppressive and regulatory function. There is an inverse relationship between testosterone and autoimmune diseases: the higher the testosterone levels, the lower the likelihood of such conditions.

See also:
- Appendix 1 ➤ Figure 7.1
- Key 4 ➤ Strengthening the Core and Abdominal Muscles

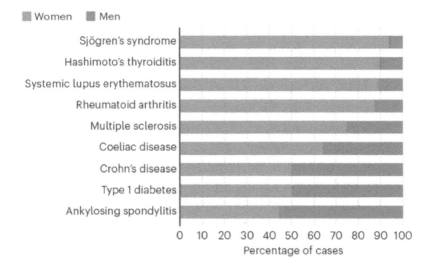

Appendix 1: Figure 7.1 - Autoimmune diseases prevalence: Males and Females

TESTOSTERONE

Generally known as the male hormone, testosterone levels are 15-20 times higher in men than in women. After the age of 30, men experience a roughly 1% drop in testosterone levels annually. Interestingly, though, this decline plateaus at age 70.

Recent research has uncovered a worrying trend. Over the last few decades, there has been a pronounced drop in testosterone levels across the population. The studies suggest that the downturn is mostly due to our modern, unhealthy lifestyle.

What are the consequences of this hormonal drop? Beyond its association with men's health, testosterone is vital for our overall well-being, affecting several aspects, from mental health to immune function. Therefore, although normal ranges differ between men and women, both genders benefit from optimizing testosterone levels.

Many of the following actionable steps used to boost your testosterone and regulate your immune system have already been discussed in other 5R+ tactics. They include:

- **Physical Exercises**: Certain workouts help improve testosterone production.
- **Prioritize Sleep**: Quality sleep is crucial.
- **Practice Contrast Showers**
- **Address Obesity**: The effects of obesity run deeper than your appearance; it is a serious *metabolic disease*. While diet is a key component of weight management, the *composition* of your gut microbiome also plays a pivotal role in regulating your weight and metabolism. The nutritional guidelines in this book naturally guide you toward achieving a healthy *BMI (Body Mass Index)*. Thus, the 5R+ system not only restores immune health but also aids in weight normalization.
- **Consume Essential Nutrients**: Ensure adequate intake of Vitamin D, Zinc, and Magnesium. The importance of these supplements has already been mentioned in relation to other DILL+ factors.
- **Other Dietary Recommendations**:
  - Increase your intake of *omega-3 (N-3)* oils.
  - Limit omega-6 *(N-6)* oils and avoid hydrogenated oils and trans fats. These are known to suppress testosterone production.
  - Reduce carbohydrate intake.

The dietary points have already been covered in Key 2, where we focused on inflammation reduction. The consistency of natural health principles across different aspects of our well-being is, indeed, fascinating!

Practices that improve your testosterone levels also fortify your overall health.

See also:

- Key 5 ➤ Exercises for Healthy Testosterone Levels
- Key 5 ➤ Sleep and Circadian Rhythms
- Key 5 ➤ Contrast Showers: A Practice You Can Start Today
- Key 2 ➤ Supplements and Inflammation
- Key 2 ➤ Inflammatory Foods

XENOESTROGENS

Some hormones significantly impact the immune system. For instance, *estrogen*, a female sex hormone, is known to increase antibody production. This effect is one reason autoimmune diseases are more commonly seen in women than in men.

In the plant world, substances like *xenoestrogens* or *phytoestrogens* mimic estrogen. They have a similar molecular structure and affect the immune system in the same way as estrogen does.

Many plant foods contain traces of phytoestrogens. However, soy has the most by far. By some estimates, the phytoestrogen content of soy is around 170 mg/kg, while its closest competitor, chickpeas, has only about 6 mg/kg. This is a key consideration for vegans leaning heavily on soy for protein. Dialing back on soy or skipping it altogether can prevent potential issues. Thankfully, there's a wide range of other plant protein sources that don't carry the same baggage.

Another product high in phytoestrogens is soy infant formula. It may have up to 190 mg/kg of phytoestrogens, compared to the much lower 0.6 mg/kg in non-soy formulas—a level specialists still consider too high for infants. The possible effects this could have, especially on reproductive health, demand further investigation.

In the same way, hormones in our food supply, from meat to dairy, can also influence immunity. Choose animal products free from added hormones and antibiotics.

Oral contraceptives are another source of hormonal disruption. Research suggests a link between their use and an increased risk of developing *Inflammatory Bowel Disease (IBD)* in women—a risk that drops after stopping the contraceptives.

See also:

• Key 2 ➤ Inflammatory Foods

PHYSICAL EXERCISES

The mere thought of physical exercise is daunting for many people dealing with autoimmune inflammation. Stiff, aching joints and tendons make movement challenging, causing intense pain. Adding fuel to the fire, misguided activities can cause harm and aggravate your condition. Nevertheless, there are usually safe ways to integrate a workout routine to improve your health.

Specific exercises play a pivotal role in our 5R+ system. Done correctly, they effectively address the DILL+ locks of the primary disease. This chapter will outline the principles of safe workouts for those with autoimmune inflammation. The process is progressive: as your condition improves, you can incrementally intensify your routine. However, always listen to your body; ease off if an exercise causes pain or strains your joints excessively. With active inflammation, always stay within your comfort zone.

It can't be stressed enough: consult with your healthcare practitioner. They can help you identify any specific limitations you may have.

TIMING

Before exploring specific practices, it's essential to remember one fundamental rule:

Never exercise on a full stomach.

After a meal, blood flow to the gut increases to support the digestion of your food. When you do intense physical activity, blood is diverted to the muscles as they need more oxygen and nutrients for work. So, exercising after a meal creates a "conflict of interests" within your body. While this may not trouble a healthy person, it is detrimental for someone with intestinal inflammation or a disrupted gut microbiome. The already compromised and sensitive gut lining receives less oxygen during digestion and absorption and is easily damaged. This worsens conditions such as *Leaky Gut* and slows down the epithelium's healing.

When is the ideal time to exercise after eating? It is best to wait 1-2 hours after consuming fruits and 4-6 hours after more substantial protein-rich meals, especially meat. This is why the best times are typically early mornings, before breakfast, or evenings if you adopt a reduced meal frequency and avoid eating after midday.

See also:

• Key 3 ➢ Obstacle #8: Snacking and Frequent Meals

EXERCISES FOR HEALTHY TESTOSTERONE LEVELS

Healthy testosterone levels are essential for immune system regulation in both males and females, as highlighted in the previous chapter. While some forms of exercise benefit testosterone production, others may suppress it.

> High-Intensity Interval Training (HIIT) is a form of exercise consisting of short bursts of intense activity alternated with brief periods of rest or lower-intensity exercise. Typically, a HIIT session involves 30-60 seconds of hard rowing, sprinting, cycling, or bodyweight exercises such as burpees or push-ups, followed by 1-2 minutes of walking or complete rest. This cycle is repeated several times, usually for 20-30 minutes.

Strength training and *high-intensity interval training (HIIT)* are potent allies, rapidly increasing your testosterone levels. In contrast, cardio activities do not provide the same improvement even though they have other health benefits. Endurance exercises like long-distance running and cycling may even lower testosterone.

Exercises that work the large muscle groups in the lower body offer the best testosterone-enhancing effects. Simple arm workouts are not enough. The most effective exercises are done with weights and include:

- Squats
- Deadlifts
- Bench presses
- Weightlifting
- Rows
- Lunges

If you enjoy running, cycling, or swimming, focus on brief, intense sessions or *HIIT*. Such explosive, short activities are known to raise testosterone levels. On the other hand, extended endurance exercises trigger the release of stress hormones, which can cause a drop in testosterone.

Keep cardio workouts to no more than 30 minutes. Although longer sessions boost stamina, they over-strain joints, cause inflammation, and are unlikely to increase testosterone levels. Marathon runners often see a substantial testosterone decrease post-race, though it does recover later. Similarly, male swimmers undertaking intense endurance training have lower testosterone concentrations.

Swimming is undeniably a fantastic workout, but there's a catch. Chlorine, typically used to keep pool water clean, has adverse health effects. Of particular concern are indoor pools where chlorine concentration in the air above the pool is higher and inhaled more directly. Research shows that regularly swimming in such pools during childhood is associated with an increased risk of certain allergies and reduced testosterone levels. It is better to use well-ventilated outdoor pools or those where ozonation, ionization, or UV water treatment are used as they have substantially lower chlorine levels. Better still is swimming in the sea or clean natural reservoirs where chlorine isn't a concern.

CORE AND ABDOMINAL MUSCLES

Strengthening your core and abdominal muscles is essential for maintaining healthy tone and motility in the digestive system. This helps to combat the *Lazy Gut* DILL+ factor, as we covered in Key 4.

See also:
- Key 4 ➤ Strengthening the Core and Abdominal Muscles
- Appendix 1 ➤ Video guides 6.3, 6.4

MUSCLE STRENGTH AND JOINTS

With autoimmune inflammation, such as arthritis, joints are often the primary areas of concern. Strengthening the muscles around them reduces the strain on the joint cartilage—it slows wear and aids healing. However, exercising inflamed joints can increase inflammation if not done correctly. Thus, achieving the right balance is crucial. You need to build stronger muscles to support your joints, but you need to do so without placing additional stress on them. Several effective tactics can help:

- Incorporate *Pilates* and other stretching exercises. The slow, deliberate movements in these practices protect the cartilage.
- Choose exercises that involve *pulling* weight rather than *pushing* it, such as incline rows, inverted rows, and pull-ups. Even hanging from a bar can significantly strengthen the arms and back. All these activities build muscle strength without exerting direct pressure on the joints.
- Use a stationary bicycle, rowing machine, or an elliptical machine for cardiovascular and strength benefits. Unlike running or walking, they cause minimal joint stress.
- Swimming is an excellent form of resistance movement,

exercising numerous muscle groups while being easy on joints.

 The key is to exercise muscles without exerting pressure on your joints.

Maintaining joint motion without added pressure is essential to heal and preserve joint health. If you can't do "real workouts," incorporate gentle stretching, moderate active or passive movements, and massage into your daily routine instead. All activity, no matter how light, is always better than none.

EXERCISE HANGOVER

Remember, feeling better and without pain is not a green light to push your boundaries. At this point, overloading your joints with strenuous activities such as going on a long hike can aggravate your condition. I know first-hand what it's like. There have been times when I've enthusiastically embraced the sense of wellness, neglected my arthritis, and tackled extensive outdoor trails, only to be crippled by pain the next day—so much so that getting out of bed was impossible. I refer to this delayed suffering as the *"exercise hangover."*

Be cautious and patient in your activities. Healing from a decade-long ailment doesn't happen overnight. It may take a year or two before your joints can endure the same stress as those of a healthy person without the backlash of inflammation. Progress slowly and be prepared to take a step back when necessary. The old Latin adage *"Festina lente,"* meaning "make haste slowly," applies perfectly here.

It is similar to the *"Eliminate-Reintroduce-Reset Technique (ERR)"* for gut health we discussed in *Key 3*. In a nutshell: it is a gradual dietary expansion, starting with well-tolerated foods, then slowly adding new ones and monitoring your body's response. If there is no negative reaction, you can go on and try something else. When it doesn't go well, you take a step back and allow your gut time to *Reset*.

Use the same approach for physical activities. Start with short workouts, focusing on gentle exercises, tracking your progress and symptoms, and allowing enough time to recover between workouts. Just as your intestinal epithelium needs time to heal, your joints, tendons, and muscles require an extended recovery time. In general, your tissues require more time to recuperate than those of a person in full health. So, start slowly, and don't be tempted to rush the process—extend your recovery time as necessary. When needed, allow several rest days between workouts to allow inflammation to diminish, similar to the dietary "*Reset*," where water fasting can help reduce inflammation.

 Festina lente. Gradual and cautious steps are the quickest path to recovery.

IMPROVE BLOOD CIRCULATION IN YOUR LIMBS: A SIMPLE EXERCISE

In my quest to overcome the misery of "*exercise hangovers*," I experimented with various exercises and improvised movements. I was searching for an activity that improves lymph drainage and blood flow through the capillaries, reducing swelling and inflammation in the arms and legs. Through trial and error, I found a simple routine, later discovering it closely mirrored a technique by Katsudzo Nishi, a renowned Japanese health teacher. You may also find other exercises from Nishi's System helpful, particularly those targeting spinal health.

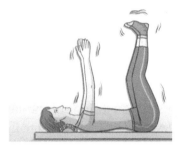

Appendix 1: Video 7.2 - Nishi Shiki, Capillary circulation exercise. Video Guide.

Here's how to perform the exercise (see **Appendix 1** for a video demonstration):

1. Begin by lying on a firm, flat surface.
2. Raise your legs and arms toward the ceiling, keeping your knees and elbows slightly bent.

3. Allow your body to relax as you give your limbs an intense, vibratory shake for several minutes.

It's the vibratory motion that's essential here—aim for a steady, moderate range of movement at a brisk pace. There are many ways to do this exercise. Experiment with various rhythms and motion patterns to find one that suits you. I found the "volleyball" pattern most effective—imagine batting away a barrage of volleyballs with both arms and legs in unison. Make sure to engage every joint in the motion, stretching and flexing from your ankles and toes up to your knees and from your fingers to your elbows. This dynamic movement promotes improved blood and lymph circulation and can be a vital part of your wellness routine.

See also:

• Appendix 1 ➢ Video 7.2

CARDIO TRAINING

Excessive exercise can aggravate intestinal epithelium damage and leaky gut syndrome. During intense workouts, your body temperature rises, blood flow to the intestines is reduced, and blood glutamine levels may drop, potentially affecting your gut health. For a healthy person, this disruption is temporary and harmless. However, if you're battling chronic inflammation, a workout like this may worsen the problem.

On the other hand, moderate cardio exercise is beneficial—it supports the immune system and enhances digestive health.

Follow these guidelines to reap the benefits of exercise without the adverse effects:

• **Exercise Duration**: Moderate the length of your workouts according to your capabilities. 20-25 minutes is often best, but if you're dealing with *IBS*, *IBD*, or *Crohn's*, even shorter workouts are better. Start with 10 minutes and increase cautiously—only as your intestinal lining health improves.

- **Timing**: As we already mentioned, avoid exercising shortly after meals. Reducing blood flow to the gut when food is present can harm the already vulnerable epithelium.
- **Consider Glutamine Supplements**: On the days you work out, glutamine supplements can support gut lining health.
- **Choose Joint-Friendly Cardio**: Since your joints absorb the pressure of your full weight with each step when running and walking, opt for alternative exercises that don't stress them. Good options are cycling, swimming, rowing, or using an elliptical machine.
- **Mind Your Weight**: If you're managing obesity, postpone running and long walks until your weight reaches a healthy range.
- **Swim for Muscle and Joint Health**: Moderate-distance swimming is an excellent workout that strengthens muscles with minimal joint impact. It's particularly beneficial if you suffer from vertebral joint inflammation, as it strengthens the spinal muscles that support the joints.

See also:
- Key 3 ➤ Active Repair ➤ Other Nutrients ➤ Glutamine

SLEEP AND CIRCADIAN RHYTHMS

SLEEP'S ROLE IN COMBATING CHRONIC ILLNESS

Don't underestimate the risks of sleep deprivation. Although often overlooked, it is a significant contributor to chronic diseases and has a complex relationship with autoimmune disorders. It causes a surge of pro-inflammatory *cytokines*, raises inflammation markers like *C-reactive protein*, and silently exacerbates chronic inflammation, increasing pain. To make matters worse, lack of sleep also impairs your immune system's ability to fend off infections. Amongst other issues, this combined effect weakens the gut's defense barrier, contributing to chronic intestinal inflammation and *Leaky Gut* conditions—two critical factors in the DILL+ scenario.

As mentioned before, gut epithelium regeneration is most active while you sleep. These critical recovery processes, as well as testosterone production, are impaired when you don't get enough rest, further damaging intestinal health and disrupting immune regulation.

The link between sleeplessness and autoimmune conditions is a two-way street. Just as insufficient slumber affects your physical and mental well-being, so the persistent pain of many autoimmune conditions makes it difficult to get a good night's rest. Thus, as you gradually reduce inflammation, you can look forward to better-quality sleep.

So, how much sleep do you need? It depends on your life stage—adults need less than children and teens. It is also affected by the season—we should sleep about two hours more in winter than in summer. The goal is to wake up on your own rather than being jolted awake by an alarm. If you have to rely on piercing sound to rouse you and waking is difficult, you are not getting enough rest. Upon rising, you should feel refreshed and ready to tackle the day. If you often feel tired and struggle to stay alert throughout the day, adjust your routine by going to bed earlier rather than sleeping in, aligning with your natural *circadian rhythms*.

See also:

• Key 5 ➤ Testosterone

Age Group		Recommended Hours of Sleep Per Day
Newborn	0-3 months	14-17 hours
Infant	4-12 months	12-16 hours
Toddler	1-2 years	11-14 hours
Preschool	3-5 years	10-13 hours
School Age	6-12 years	9-12 hours
Teen	13-18 months	8-10 hours
Adult	18-64 years	7-9 hours
	65 years and older	7-8 hours

Appendix 1: Table 7.3 - Recommended Hours of Sleep Per Day. Source: Centers for Disease Control and Prevention

CIRCADIAN RHYTHMS

 Early to bed and early to rise. ~ Benjamin Franklin

When you sleep is almost as important as how much you sleep. Many physiological processes follow natural day-night and seasonal cycles, known as *circadian rhythms*. They ensure the proper working of all body systems and can also affect disease activity.

> Daily circadian rhythms are natural cycles influenced by light. Over 24 hours, they coordinate a range of bodily functions, including sleep, wakefulness, body temperature regulation, hormone production, digestion, regeneration, and more. Disruptions in circadian rhythms affect metabolism, the immune system, and cognitive abilities, profoundly impacting overall health. This is why jet lag, shift work, sleep deprivation, or late bedtime patterns lead to significant health problems.

If you are living with *Rheumatoid Arthritis (RA)*, you are likely familiar with *morning joint stiffness*. This is just one example of these cyclical body functions. The morning *interleukin IL-6* production, which drives this inflammation, can be almost ten times higher than normal in people with RA. Later in the day, the production of the hormone *cortisol* follows its daily cycle, reducing inflammation and bringing relief. Morning joint stiffness is a tangible manifestation of how your body's internal rhythms affect chronic illness. However, not all effects of circadian rhythms are immediately noticeable. Two processes central to healing the autoimmune DILL+ factors—digestive system restoration and epithelial lining regeneration—aren't obvious to your senses. Yet, their changes ripple through the entire body.

The same is true for your body's ecosystem and microbiome. Because we all live under the same sun, the ebb and flow of 24-hour and seasonal cycles affect all life forms, big and small. Research shows that your body's rhythms, including disrupted sleep patterns, can have a cascading effect on your gut bacteria and vice versa.

Sleep's place in the daily cycle should not be changed. For millennia, midnight signified the middle of the night, a time for sleep, while noon marked the middle of the day. With no form of artificial light, our ancestors typically went to sleep shortly after sunset and woke up before sunrise.

In ancient Rome, government officials started work before sunrise

—around 5-6 a.m.—and concluded their business at noon. Most people followed a similar schedule, winding down their workday by noon and reserving afternoons for leisure with family and friends. Often, a nap was taken, a practice now known as the Spanish "siesta." It was initially a post-work activity rather than a mid-work pause.

In an entirely different culture and geography, the Middle East, traditional Muslim prayers reflect a similar schedule. The earliest prayer is at dawn, before sunrise (5-6 a.m.), while the final prayer of the day, called the nighttime prayer, occurs right after sunset (7-9 p.m.). Nowadays, few modern people consider 7 p.m. nighttime, never mind bedtime. This pattern of living according to the sun's cycle and circadian rhythms is a common thread across traditional cultures. These routines were not ruled by a fixed time schedule. Rather, they were adjusted seasonally, aligning with the changes in sunlight. Today, we recognize the medical importance of this practice. In winter, when we have fewer sunlight hours, our bodies require more sleep—an extra 1.5 to 2.5 hours—compared to summer.

 We should regularly observe both sunrise and sunset.

Modern lifestyles, artificial lighting, and screens of all sizes, from TVs to phones, have significantly disrupted our sleep patterns and daily circadian rhythms, taking a toll on our health. This increasingly common societal shift, introduced to children from an early age, often becomes a deeply ingrained habit. People who adapt to this lifestyle are referred to as "night owls"—they prefer being active late into the evening and sleeping in. Changing such a lifelong practice and returning to normal sleep patterns—according to circadian rhythms— is paramount to good health, but it takes time.

 Common does not mean normal!

Even if the demands of the modern world prevent you from adopting your ancestors' sleep schedule, you can improve your own by following these simple rules:

- Aim to be in bed by 9 p.m.
- Stop consuming caffeine and other stimulants at least six hours before going to sleep. Even better: avoid them completely.
- Refrain from eating for four hours before retiring for the night.
- Avoid screen time for at least two hours before bedtime (more on this later).
- Do moderate physical activity, preferably outdoors, to enhance your sleep quality.

An early bedtime means you will naturally wake up earlier, eliminating the need for an alarm clock and giving yourself ample time for tasks you might have previously done in the late evening.

Sleep Cycle Disruption

Sleep is not simply one long, uniform period of rest; it is a series of complex brain activity cycles, each lasting about 90 to 110 minutes. Typically, you'll go through four to six of these cycles each night, ideally waking naturally at the end of the last one. Herein lies the problem with alarm clocks: they jolt you awake mid-cycle, disrupting your natural sleep structure, diminishing its effectiveness, and raising your risk of developing a range of health issues.

There is a smarter approach for those times when an alarm is necessary. You can download one of the mobile apps that track your sleep phases by analyzing your breathing patterns. Instead of a fixed-time alarm that disrupts your natural sleep structure, set up your app to sound the alarm close to your desired time but coinciding with the end of a sleep cycle. The apps often also include features to analyze overall sleep quality, such as monitoring snoring, bedtime habits, ambient noise, etc. See app recommendations in *Appendix 1*.

See also:

- Appendix 1 ➢ Table 7.5

· · ·

SCREENS, BULBS, AND NIGHT LIGHT

A special note of caution: The blue light emitted by devices such as TVs, phones, and computers interferes with the production of melatonin, a hormone responsible for making you sleepy.

For a smooth transition to sleep, aim to eliminate screen time 1-2 hours before bedtime. Replace these activities with moderate physical exercise—ideally outdoors, though indoors is also fine—and consider reading as a calming pre-sleep ritual. If you read ebooks, choose an e-reader with an e-ink screen that doesn't emit light.

Light Type	Temperature Range (Kelvin)	Applications
A candle	1800K	
Very warm, Soft	1800K - 2400K	Creating a cozy and relaxing atmosphere, ideal for bedrooms.
Warm, Soft.	2500K - 3200K	Providing a warm and inviting ambiance, suitable for bedrooms, living rooms, etc.
Neutral, Cool white	3300K - 4000K	Promoting alertness and focus, perfect for kitchens, bathrooms, home offices, etc.
Daylight	4100K - 5000K	Simulating natural daylight, enhancing task performance and mood. Suitable for home offices.
Cool daylight, Natural sunlight	5500K - 6500K	Mimicking natural sunlight, ideal for areas requiring bright illumination, such as workshops.
Blue sky	10000K	

Appendix 1: Table 7.4 - Light temperature range and applications

If working on a screen in the evening is unavoidable, reduce its impact by adjusting your device's light settings. Many platforms now offer this option under the name "Night Light," "Night Shift Mode," or "Reduced Blue Light." These settings adjust your screen's light spectrum to emit softer, lower-frequency light similar to the natural glow of the evening sky, making screens less disruptive to your circadian rhythms. For best results, set all your devices to automatically switch to this mode from just before sunset until sunrise.

Similarly, electric light in modern houses can significantly disrupt healthy sleep. Fortunately, this issue is easily remedied by choosing light bulbs that emit a softer, warmer glow, as measured by light temperature grades. Strategically install bulbs in your home, using neutral or cooler light for your daytime work areas, warmer light for evening relaxation spaces, and "soft," low-temperature light bulbs in your bedroom to create a sleep-conducive environment.

See also:

• Appendix 1 ➢ Table 7.4

MELATONIN: FRIEND OR FOE?

> Melatonin is a hormone produced by the brain's pineal gland in response to darkness. It regulates daily and seasonal circadian rhythms and plays other vital roles, including moderating the immune system. Exposure to light at night, even during sleep, can suppress melatonin production.

Few hormones have caught the attention of supplement manufacturers like *melatonin*. Sleep aids containing this circadian rhythm-regulating hormone have become popular go-tos for people seeking better sleep and health. However, more thorough research is needed to establish their safety and effectiveness. This is especially critical for autoimmune diseases, as the impact of melatonin on such conditions is complex. I usually recommend against using melatonin supplements. Instead, focus on normalizing the body's natural hormone production through healthy sleep habits.

Indeed, melatonin plays a role in regulating the immune system, but research presents a mixed picture. It can be beneficial in some instances, but in others, such as arthritis and multiple sclerosis, it may worsen the autoimmune condition. Such varied outcomes occur due to melatonin's effects on several factors through different pathways. On the one hand, it can boost the immune response, increasing existing inflammation. On the other hand, it promotes gut lining repair, strengthening the protective barrier against *Leaky Gut*, which is helpful in conditions such as *IBS* or *Crohn's* disease. Thus, melatonin impacts various DILL+ aspects differently.

In addition, some studies suggest that normalizing melatonin production can help prevent migraine pain.

VITAMIN D AND MELATONIN

The sunshine vitamin—vitamin D—is synthesized when your skin is exposed to sunlight. Conversely, melatonin production occurs in darkness. This inverse relationship implies that a shift in the balance between light and darkness stimulates the production of one while suppressing the other. Living in northern countries, which experience reduced sunlight exposure, can significantly increase melatonin levels and decrease vitamin D. This contributes to the higher prevalence of autoimmune diseases in higher latitudes.

Hence, it is crucial to consider the ratio of vitamin D and melatonin concentrations, along with natural circadian rhythms in melatonin production. Taking melatonin supplements can disrupt this delicate balance. Therefore, as mentioned before, the safer approach is to support your body's natural processes.

Increase your sunlight exposure, especially in winter and in regions with limited daylight. In such areas, cool daylight bulbs (5500K-6500K) are invaluable tools for mimicking natural sunlight. Remember, this should be restricted to daytime hours only.

In addition to increased daylight exposure, ensure your sleep environment is dark for optimal melatonin production. Research has shown that the pineal gland can detect light even through closed eyelids during certain sleep phases, affecting melatonin synthesis.

 We need a sharp contrast between bright sunlight and inky darkness in our day-night cycles.

Lastly, ensure adequate Vitamin D intake through supplements, especially in winter and if you spend extended periods indoors.

See also:

• Key 2 ➤ Supplements and Inflammation ➤ Vitamin D

SNORING AND SLEEP APNEA: HIDDEN THREATS TO BRAIN HEALTH

Sleep quality matters as much as quantity: it isn't only about how long and when you sleep, but also how well you sleep.

A common disruptor of sleep quality is snoring. This noisy bedtime breathing isn't merely an annoyance; it can lead to a chronic lack of oxygen during sleep. In severe cases, breathing might even stop for up to a minute, causing the suffocating brain to jolt awake, often with a snort or a gasp. This constant battle against oxygen deprivation disrupts your sleep cycle and may lead to brain injury and overall bodily harm. Such extreme cases are referred to as *sleep apnea* and demand immediate medical intervention.

However, even less severe snoring, persisting over months or years, takes a toll on your body. Besides other harmful effects, connections to immune disorders have been found. Here are the most obvious signs of the problem:

- **Reported snoring or breathing pauses:** Your spouse can likely tell you if you snore or experience a pause between breaths while you sleep.
- **Restless sleep, gasping, or choking at night:** When your brain doesn't get enough oxygen during sleep, it rouses you, disrupting your sleep.
- **Excessive daytime sleepiness and difficulty concentrating:** Snoring causes repeated sleep interruptions, reducing the amount of deep sleep necessary for the brain to recover. This leads to brain fog and drowsiness during the day.
- **Morning headaches:** Oxygen starvation can result in headaches upon waking, indicating potential harm to brain cells.

- **Sore throat upon awakening:** Snoring causes turbulent airflow and, thus, irritation in the throat. It also makes your airways more susceptible to infections.
- **Chest pain at night:** Oxygen deprivation is harmful not only to the brain but also to the heart.
- **High blood pressure:** Sometimes, snoring is the hidden cause of *hypertension*, and addressing it can help resolve the condition.

Family members might alert you to your nighttime breathing issues, but specialized mobile apps can monitor your sleep more precisely. Some apps can track sleep cycles, record sleep sounds, and indicate snoring or sleep apnea. See **Appendix 1** for recommendations.

What you can do:

- **Avoid alcohol and drugs:** These substances can aggravate snoring.
- **Adjust your sleep position:** Sleeping on your back often worsens snoring due to gravity's effect on the throat and tongue. Try sleeping on your side or stomach, and use a smaller, firmer pillow.
- **Address obesity:** Being overweight increases the likelihood of snoring because excess throat tissue easily blocks airflow. Follow the strategies in this book to normalize your weight gradually.
- **Strengthen throat and tongue muscles:** The next section discusses *Oropharyngeal Exercises* for this purpose.

If these measures don't yield results, consult a doctor. They might recommend:

- **Oral appliances:** Devices worn in the mouth during sleep to keep airways open.
- *CPAP (Continuous Positive Airway Pressure)* **Machine:** A device that uses air pressure to keep your airways open during sleep.

- **Surgery:** In some cases, this might be a necessary option.

Every year, I research the latest tools for addressing sleep problems and share my findings with my subscribers. To access this annual report, join our community at www.autoimmunityunlocked.org.

See also:
- Appendix 1 ➤ Table 7.5

Oropharyngeal Exercises

As you transition from light to deep sleep, the muscles in your throat, tongue, and the roof of your mouth (*soft palate*) relax. This relaxation can cause these tissues to partially block your airway, resulting in vibrations that produce the snoring sound. In severe cases, the airway may become completely blocked, leading to pauses in breathing, known as *sleep apnea*. Sensing this oxygen deprivation, the brain is partially roused, prompting you to reposition, clear the obstruction, and resume breathing.

This is why it is critical to improve muscle tone in these areas. Stronger muscles in your throat and soft palate can prevent them from collapsing and obstructing your airway. Similarly, your tongue is less likely to fall back and block airflow if it has good muscle tone. Thus, strength in these tissues reduces snoring and enhances your overall sleep quality and health. It can be achieved by doing specific *Oropharyngeal Exercises*. Follow the guidelines in the videos in **Appendix 1**.

See also:
- Appendix 1 ➤ Video guides 7.6, 7.7, 7.8

YOUR DIGESTIVE SYSTEM ALSO WANTS TO SLEEP

In our journey to resolve autoimmune conditions, we've uncovered a crucial link: restoration of the *microbiome*, *gut epithelium*, and *motility* are vital for the immune system. This is why, among all the body's circadian rhythms, those governing the digestive system are especially important.

Similar to sleep, your digestive system follows a natural day-night rhythm. Typically, *peristalsis* (wave-like muscle contractions that move food through the digestive system) and digestive juice production are suppressed a couple of hours after sunset. This starts the gut's night rest period, regardless of your personal schedule. Ideally, no active digestion should be initiated in the last two hours before sunset.

 No night shifts for your alimentary tract.

As previously discussed, digestive juices and strong intestinal motility are essential for maintaining a healthy intestine, microbiome, and immune system. Introducing food into the digestive tract just before its "close of business" feeds pathogenic bacteria, increases inflammation, and allows partially digested molecules to leak into the bloodstream—all detrimental DILL+ factors covered in *Keys 1-4*.

You can't sleep and work at the same time. The same principle applies to your intestine.

During sleep, your body prioritizes critical regeneration processes, such as repairing the gut epithelium. Because digestion disrupts this "maintenance time," hunger intervals are crucial for treating leaky gut, as discussed in Key 3. The most important of these extended hunger intervals is nighttime, while you are asleep.

It's better to go to bed hungry and wake up with a healthier appetite in the morning than to satiate your appetite before retiring for the night.

 Do not sabotage the nightly repair work.

Follow a simple rule of thumb: no food, tea, coffee, or calorie-containing beverages for 3 hours before bedtime. If your meal includes protein-rich foods, especially meat, extend this to 4-6 hours. Should you feel the urge to eat in the evening, choose fruits, as they digest quickly and easily, and ensure you maintain the 3-hour window before retiring for the night. Save heavier meals for the first half of the day.

Aligning your eating habits with your body's natural rhythms not only aids in gut repair but also enhances the quality of your sleep and reduces the risk of snoring. Moreover, it's a proactive measure against *heartburn (gastroesophageal reflux).*

See also:

- Key 3 ➢ Obstacle #8: Snacking and Frequent Meals
- Key 1 ➢ Stomach Acid ➢ Antacids and "Heartburn" (Gastroesophageal Reflux)

HYDROTHERAPY AND TEMPERATURE CONTRAST

WARM WATER: ARTHRITIS RELIEF

If you live with one of the hundreds of conditions that cause inflamed joints and muscles, you've probably experienced the soothing relief of a warm bath or shower. Due to water's conductivity, it transmits warmth deep into your body, enhancing blood flow to stiff muscles and joints, which helps loosen them and alleviate pain, promoting smoother movement. The heat also softens thickened *synovial fluid*, the lubricant in your joints, easing movement and reducing inflammation.

In addition, submerging your body in water takes advantage of its buoyancy, reducing joint strain and helping your muscles relax. With this gentle support, movement is easier and less painful, making water the ideal place to stretch and exercise. Warm water therapy is a natural complement to massage and stretching and can reduce morning stiffness, increase flexibility and range of motion, and even improve sleep quality.

Aquatic exercise, a form of *hydrotherapy*, involves working out in a pool. Options include water aerobics, water jogging, and, of course, swimming—an excellent, low-impact exercise for many conditions. The water's resistance builds muscle strength, while its shock-absorbing quality lessens the impact on joints.

Notes:

- It's common to experience swelling in your legs and feet after a hot shower or bath due to dilated vessels and relaxed muscles. To counteract this, consider *contrast showers*, discussed next, and exercises to enhance capillary circulation in limbs, as previously described.
- Always use water that is comfortably warm, not excessively hot.
- Prevent catching a cold after a warm bath or shower by drying yourself thoroughly. Better yet, conclude your warm session with a cold shower for 10-30 seconds, followed by thorough drying. While a few seconds of cold water won't "cool down" your body, it triggers a reflex that constricts your skin vessels to conserve heat. This also serves as a stepping stone towards contrast showers, offering more profound benefits.
- Remember, warm baths provide relief and enhance blood circulation, similar to massage and stretching, but they don't address the underlying immune system issues. However, consistently applying all 5R+ strategies does!

See also:
- Key 5 ➤ Physical Exercises
- Key 5 ➤ Physical Exercises ➤ Improve Blood Circulation in Your Limbs: A Simple Exercise

CONTRAST SHOWERS: A PRACTICE YOU CAN START TODAY

The concept of alternating hot and cold temperatures for health and well-being has deep historical roots, dating back to ancient civilizations. Traditional methods practiced in various cultures follow a similar pattern: sharp temperature contrasts and short durations—particularly for the cold phase. Ancient Greek and Roman bathhouses, and later versions in Ottoman and modern Turkish baths, commonly feature a combination of hot and cold pools. This tradition of temperature alternation is followed in more northern countries, too. For instance, the Russian *parilka* (or, *banya*) typically combines the intense heat of a steam room with the invigorating act of rubbing snow on the body. Likewise, traditional Finnish *saunas* involve extreme heat in a dry room followed by a plunge into an ice-cold pool. Nowadays, a simplified form of this ancient wellness practice can be easily emulated at home using your shower faucet to swiftly alternate between hot and cold water.

One of the key health benefits of contrast showers is the stimulation of your body's blood circulation. The initial high temperature causes blood vessels to dilate, moving blood from your core to the surface and extremities. A swift change to cold water makes these vessels constrict, pushing blood back toward the core. This dynamic 'pumping' action not only improves blood circulation but also promotes the removal of stagnant bodily waste products, thus supporting *detoxification*. It also alters tissue temperatures, eases muscle spasms, reduces inflammation, and strengthens immune function—providing an *immunomodulatory* effect.

Contrast showers have also been shown to improve sleep quality, making them an excellent routine before bedtime. They reduce the time it takes to fall asleep, providing a deeper, more restful night. The refreshing "shock" of the cold phase benefits the nervous system and has been linked to increased testosterone levels, boosting overall vitality.

Finally, this practice can also significantly reduce platelet stickiness and aggregation, lowering the risk of dangerous blood clot formation. This is particularly beneficial for those with *cardiovascular* issues, such as *ischemic heart disease*.

Start gradually. For contrast showers, 'gradual' refers to time, not temperature. The initial duration of cold exposure can be just a few seconds, yet it should be really cold. Keep the cold phase under 30 seconds to ensure that only your skin's surface is cooled and the chill does not penetrate your body. Instead, it drives blood to your core and increases the temperature of your internal organs. This is why pouring cold water on a person suffering from heatstroke can be dangerous; a lukewarm temperature should be used!

Aim for a brief cold shock without losing your body's heat.

Here's a step-by-step guide for contrast showers:

- Begin your shower with warm water, adjusting it to a comfortable level.
- After a few minutes, increase the temperature to the hottest you can reasonably endure for 2-3 minutes.
- Next, switch the temperature to as cold as you can stand for about 10 seconds.
- Alternate between hot and cold for 3-5 cycles.
- Over several weeks, as you become more accustomed, gradually extend the cold exposure up to 30 seconds. Increasing the hot phase duration beyond 3 minutes is not necessary.
- Always complete your final cycle with cold water to tighten skin vessels, close pores, and reduce any swelling.
- After exiting the shower, dry yourself thoroughly with a towel to retain warmth and prevent catching a cold.

Caution: Avoid prolonged exposure to cold water, as it increases the risk of hypothermia. You can decrease the temperature for greater contrast but keep the exposure brief.

SAUNA AND STEAM ROOM

Building upon the health effects of contrast showers, let's explore the benefits of *saunas* (dry heat rooms) and *steam rooms* (high humidity heat rooms). These are powerful tools in your arsenal against pain and chronic inflammation. They work similarly to contrast showers but have more pronounced effects due to higher temperatures and longer heat exposure.

Key Benefits:

- **Detoxification:** Profuse perspiration effectively removes toxins from your body, which helps manage chronic inflammation and infections.
- **Muscle Relaxation and Pain Relief:** The intense heat deeply penetrates your muscles, easing arthritis stiffness and pain. For enhanced effectiveness, practice stretching and massaging inflamed joints in the sauna.
- **Immunity:** Regular sauna sessions have been shown to improve immune system functions.
- **Cardiovascular Health:** The high temperature dilates blood vessels and boosts blood flow throughout the body. Your heart has to work harder to pump your blood through the widened vessels, giving it a 'workout challenge' similar to cardiovascular exercise.

Warning: If you have any heart condition, proceed with care, gradually increasing the time in the heat room. Always consult your doctor before starting.

Regimen: Finnish studies recommend spending 15-30 minutes in a sauna, set between 70-100°C (160-210°F), two to four times a week. For steam rooms, with their high humidity, the temperature range is lower: 40-50°C (110-120°F).

Cool-Down: After each session, take a cold shower or plunge into a cold pool for 10 to 30 seconds. This practice helps close the skin pores dilated by heat and sweating, improves circulation, prevents catching a cold, and enhances the overall therapeutic effect.

 Conclude each hydrotherapy with a cold water rinse and thorough body drying.

Precautions and Preparation:

- **Progress Slowly:** Begin with shorter sessions and gradually increase the duration of your heat room exposure over several weeks.

- **Hydration:** Drink plenty of water before and after your sauna session to replenish fluids lost through sweating.
- **Empty Stomach:** Only use the sauna when your stomach is empty. Remember from our discussion on exercise that diverting blood away from the intestines during digestion can worsen leaky gut conditions.
- **Medical Warning:** If you have any heart or blood vessel disease, exercise caution by slowly increasing your session length. Consult with your doctor before starting. Do not use saunas or steam rooms during pregnancy!

CONTRAINDICATIONS AND WARNINGS

The described hydrotherapy techniques are powerful tools for managing a range of conditions, including autoimmune diseases. They support immune and cardiovascular health, and promote the removal of toxins from the body.

However, as with any potent therapeutic approach, some people should use these methods with caution, and others must avoid them altogether. Consult with your doctor to understand what is safe for your particular situation.

Here is a non-exhaustive list of conditions where consulting with your doctor is especially important:

- Pregnancy, particularly if temperature exceeds 35°C (95°F).
- Acute infections.
- Recent injuries (within 48 hours).
- Open wounds.
- Acute inflammation.
- Edema (swelling).
- Bleeding disorders.
- Peripheral vascular disease.
- Localized cancer.
- Neuropathy (impaired sensation).
- Impaired communication ability.
- Recent cerebral hemorrhage (within three weeks).

- Epilepsy.
- Cognitive impairments, such as dementia.
- Diabetes, particularly with neuropathy or peripheral vascular disease.
- Acute vomiting or diarrhea.
- Allergy to chlorine or bromine used in pool maintenance.
- Shortness of breath at rest.
- Uncontrolled cardiac failure or paroxysmal nocturnal dyspnea (sudden shortness of breath during sleep).
- Resting or unstable angina.
- Known aneurysm.
- HIV and Hepatitis C (advised not to enter the pool during menstruation).
- Obesity, which may present challenges during water rescues.

ELIMINATE OTHER AUTOIMMUNE TRIGGERS

CHRONIC INFLAMMATION IN YOUR BODY

Inflammation is your body's natural response to infection or trauma, a battle between your immune cells and the intruder, normally culminating quickly in a decisive victory: healing. However, in some cases, this process transforms into a "cold war," a protracted conflict lasting months or even years. It becomes *chronic inflammation*, progressively harming your body and undermining your health.

In *Key 2*, we explored how chronic inflammation can exhaust the immune system and lead to errors, setting the stage for autoimmune diseases and allergies. A classic example is rheumatic fever, one of the first described autoimmune conditions linked to chronic infection. Numerous other infections can also act as triggers, including *Epstein-Barr* virus, *Proteus*, *Chlamydia*, *Pneumococcus*, etc.

Chronic inflammation in the intestine is the biggest concern, especially since over half of your immune cells reside there. The widespread prevalence of unhealthy diets and disrupted microbiomes in today's world often causes this condition, which can grow undetected for a long time, making it more problematic.

However, the risk of chronic inflammation isn't confined to a single body part. It can occur in the lungs, kidneys, or other organs, often so subtly that it goes unnoticed. Symptoms such as periodically increased body temperature, transient pain, or other repeated health issues may, but not always, be a sign of its presence.

Consult with your doctor. A thorough medical checkup can help identify locations of chronic inflammation besides your main autoimmune disease. The clue sometimes lies in an illness that preceded the onset of your autoimmune condition. Think back to the year preceding your battle with autoimmunity. Did you have any infections, such as a stomach bug, influenza, or an issue with your kidneys? An autoimmune condition in one part of your body can be traced back to a problem in an entirely different organ or system.

Addressing chronic inflammation is vital. By eliminating it, you unburden your immune system, allowing it to recover and function more efficiently. Follow your doctor's treatment protocol for any chronic infections.

ORAL MICROBIOME, GUMS, AND TEETH

Your mouth is one of the most common sites of chronic inflammation. Fortunately, it's also one of the most visible and manageable. Therefore, habits that promote good oral and gum health have a direct impact on your autoimmune disease.

There are at least two pathways through which oral health can contribute to autoimmune conditions: *chronic inflammation* and the *oral microbiome*. These two aspects are intertwined and need to be addressed together. Let's explore each one to discover potential solutions.

Chronic Gum Inflammation and Dental Pockets

Chronic gum inflammation, usually found between teeth and in *periodontal pockets*, is a frequent yet often overlooked source of chronic inflammation. It not only threatens your dental health, potentially leading to tooth loss, but also poses a silent yet significant risk to your entire immune system.

Healthy gums tightly surround each tooth, forming a very shallow groove where they meet. However, when these grooves evolve into pockets deeper than 2mm (0.08 inches) due to destructive bacteria and inflammation, regular brushing becomes ineffective in cleaning them. Food debris and bacteria are trapped in the pockets where they decay, causing a vicious cycle: increased inflammation (*periodontitis*) causes deeper pockets, resulting in further accumulation of harmful substances.

> Periodontal pockets are gaps that form between the teeth and gums as a result of gum disease, which causes the breakdown of supporting tissue and bone. Bacteria and food particles get trapped in these pockets, leading to infection and tooth decay if not treated.

In addition to noticeable inflammation and pain, common signs of this condition include bleeding gums, particularly during vigorous tooth brushing, a persistent bad taste in the mouth, or bad breath. However, sometimes, the signs of periodontitis may be less obvious, existing 'below the waterline,' so to speak, and can be identified only during a thorough dental check-up.

Visit your dentist to check if you're facing this problem, and if you do, address it swiftly. Rigorous oral hygiene can turn the tide. Begin with *deep dental cleaning (scaling)*, followed by regular professional cleaning of periodontal pockets every 4-6 months. With consistent care, your gums can heal, allowing the pockets to shrink back to their ideal depth of 1-2 mm.

I cannot overstate the importance of healthy gums and teeth. Good oral care not only prevents tooth decay and loss but also lowers your risk of chronic inflammation and autoimmune conditions.

ORAL MICROBIOME

According to research, the oral microbiome is second only to the gut microbiome in importance for your immune system. Though much smaller, the oral microbiota houses over 10 billion bacteria across several hundred species. These microbes are continuously swallowed with food and saliva—like a constant wave of immigration moving down your alimentary tract. Thus, over time, unhealthy oral bacteria can change the microbial population downstream and undermine your stomach and gut health.

Part of the problem is the collection of food and microorganisms in *periodontal pockets*, as described in the previous section. These sites of stagnation and decay create ecosystem niches for pathogenic bacteria that consistently contaminate your food and the digestive system. Just as a flowing river has fewer pathogens than a swamp and proper room ventilation improves air quality, so effective removal of the contents of your mouth ensures good oral health.

 Stagnation welcomes harmful germs. Health thrives in movement.

Another factor is the food you provide for your oral microbiome. Foods high in starch and sugar foster an unhealthy bacterial environment, promoting periodontitis, as well as tooth decay and cavities.

 Sugar is the second worst thing you can do for your teeth after boxing without a mouthguard.

I've lost track of how many times, from different perspectives, we have consistently arrived at the same conclusion: **Avoid Sugar**.

Starch presents a similar problem, and its residues should always be thoroughly removed from your mouth after meals. Anthropologists find that cultures with low-starch diets have minimal dental cavities (*caries*). One notable historical instance was reported in the 13th century when the nomadic Tatars and Mongols conquered China. They were surprised to see the rotten teeth of Chinese peasants, who primarily consumed rice. In contrast, the steppe nomads, whose diet consisted mainly of dairy and greens, knew no such problems.

On the other hand, fiber-rich foods help maintain a clean environment and promote a healthy oral microbiome, similar to their beneficial effects in the gut. In general, the nutritional guidelines in this book support your digestive and immune systems as well as your dental health. Once again, we see how adopting natural, healthy lifestyle habits benefits multiple body systems. This contrasts sharply with many medicines, which usually help one part of the body while poisoning others.

Finally, be wary of popular mouthwashes and antibacterial toothpastes. Many have a "kill 'em all" effect, annihilating all bacteria, good and bad. As we discussed in our *Key 1* section, such weapons of mass destruction open the door for more aggressive and resistant bacterial strains. They outcompete and replace mild, beneficial bacteria while also reducing microbiota variety. Indiscriminate bacterial destruction isn't the solution. The next chapter suggests a more effective tactic.

BUILD A WINNING ORAL HEALTH ROUTINE

To maintain a healthy oral environment and microbiome, incorporate these four essential practices into your routine:

RINSE WITH WATER

Most foods contain acids that affect tooth enamel, temporarily weakening it. To avoid damaging it, don't brush your teeth immediately after eating. Instead, thoroughly rinse your mouth with lukewarm water after every meal and beverage to remove food particles and acidic residues from your teeth and gums.

MECHANICAL CLEANING

Wait 30-50 minutes to brush your teeth after rinsing to allow your tooth enamel to remineralize and regain its strength. Then, brush your teeth. Remember, the effectiveness of brushing lies in the mechanical action of the bristles rather than the toothpaste.

Pay special attention to the dental pockets, and ensure you clean both the inner and outer sides of your gums and teeth. The motion to sweep debris out of these pockets is downwards on the upper jaw and upwards on the lower jaw. To ensure you're effectively cleaning the groove where your tooth enamel meets your gum tissue, imagine sweeping dirt out of a room corner, moving it in a single, focused direction. See the illustration and video in Appendix 1.

Don't forget to clean between your teeth using your toothbrush and dental floss.

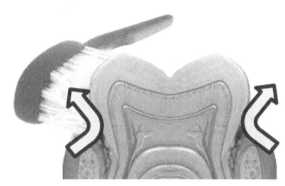

Appendix 1: Figure 7.9 - Teeth brushing direction: effective cleansing of periodontal pockets

Finally, brush your tongue from back to front, and use soft circular motions to clean the palate and insides of your cheeks to remove bacteria, decaying food particles, and dead cells.

Warning: use extra caution if you have dental crowns.

See also:

• Appendix 1 ➢ Figure 7.9, Video 7.10

Spices for Oral Microbiome

Some spices release essential oils and other beneficial compounds that improve gum health and regulate the oral microbiota. They serve as mild, natural antibacterials, curbing bacterial growth and the decay of food particles in dental pockets. This effect is similar to how spices and other products enhance the gut microbiome, as discussed in *Key 1*. The spices beneficial for oral health are:

• Bay Leaves
• Neem bark or leaves
• Clove buds

- Cardamom seeds
- Fennel seeds

Once you've finished brushing your teeth, place a few pieces of one of these spices into your mouth for 5-10 minutes. You can slowly chew them to activate the release and dispersal of their bioactive compounds throughout your mouth.

See also:

• Key 1 ➤ Feeding your Allies ➤ Good Bitter Truth

• Key 1 ➤ Other Tactics for Fixing SIBO and Normalizing Microbiome Distribution ➤ Power of Herbs, Spices, and Other Foods to Control Microbial Growth

PERIODIC PROFESSIONAL CLEANING

Regular brushing, though essential, does not efficiently remove food debris, plaque, and tartar from dental pockets deeper than 2mm. To bridge this gap, have your teeth cleaned by a dental hygienist approximately 2-3 times annually. Furthermore, consult your dentist about the need for an initial deep cleaning (scaling). These procedures complement your daily routine by targeting areas that are challenging to reach through regular brushing and flossing.

By integrating these pillars into your routine, you'll effectively maintain a healthy oral environment, protecting your teeth and gums and also helping your immune system.

✔ PRACTICAL RECAP

DILL+ Lock: + Factors Beyond Digestive Health.
5R+ Key Strategy: **R**econdition.

Below are the concise highlights of actionable steps for Key 5. For detailed information, please refer to the relevant chapters in this section.

- **Too Clean is Too Bad:**
  - Targeted Hygiene: Eliminate hazardous pathogens while increasing exposure to a diverse range of mild, common bacteria.
  - Spend more time outdoors, including dining outside.
  - Choose organically grown fruits and vegetables.
  - Avoid the "sanitizermania."
- **Environment and Climate:**
  - Address mold in your home and office, particularly in A/C systems and ducts.
  - Improve indoor air ventilation.
  - Control indoor humidity to maintain a dry environment.
  - Choose moderately sunny places over shaded ones.
  - Choose moderately warm places over cold ones.
  - Choose locations at higher elevations.

- Opt for natural airflow through open windows instead of air conditioning.
- Avoid damp, fungi-prone areas.

- **Hormonal Health:**
  - Limit exposure to xenoestrogens; consider reducing or avoiding soy products.
  - Combine strength training for large muscle groups with high-intensity interval training (HIIT).
  - Prioritize quality sleep.
  - Contrast showers.
  - Nutritional supplements: Vitamin D, Zinc, and Magnesium.
  - Address obesity.

- **Physical Exercises:**
  - Do not exercise immediately after eating.
  - Select exercises that don't strain joints:
    - Stretching and Pilates.
    - Pulling rather than pushing.
    - Moderate joint-friendly cardiovascular exercises.
  - Perform exercise that improves capillary circulation in the limbs.

- **Sleep and Circadian Rhythms:**
  - Prioritize normal sleep duration and timing.
  - Early to bed and early to rise, without an alarm.
  - Avoid eating within four hours before bedtime.
  - Avoid screen time within two hours before bedtime.
  - Use 'Night Light' settings on electronic devices to reduce blue light exposure in the evening.
  - Strategically install warm and daylight bulbs in your home.
  - Supplement with Vitamin D and normalize natural melatonin production.
  - Ensure your sleeping area is dark.
  - Address snoring and sleep apnea.
    - Perform *oropharyngeal exercises* to strengthen throat and tongue muscles.

- Seek medical help if needed.
- **Hydrotherapy and Temperature Contrast:**
  - Stretching in warm water.
  - Aquatic exercises for low-impact fitness.
  - Contrast showers or baths.
  - Sauna or steam room.
  - Finish hydrotherapy sessions with a cold rinse and thorough drying.
- **Eliminate Other Autoimmune Triggers:**
  - Identify and address any sources of chronic inflammation. Seek medical help as needed.
  - Oral Microbiome, Gums, and Teeth:
    - Address chronic gum and dental issues.
    - Sugar is a major adversary of your oral health.
    - Avoid antibacterial mouthwashes and toothpastes.
    - Rinse your mouth with water after eating or drinking.
    - Brush teeth 30-50 minutes after eating.
    - Use certain spices to improve oral microbiome.
    - Regularly undergo professional dental cleanings.

YOUR VOICE CAN TRANSFORM LIVES

Now, you have the chance to make a difference—not just for yourself, but for someone else searching for answers.

Would you lend a hand to someone who's curious about reclaiming their health but doesn't know where to begin? My mission with *Autoimmunity Unlocked* is to make transforming immune health clear, accessible, and achievable for everyone. But I can't reach everyone alone.

Most readers choose books based on reviews. By sharing your thoughts, you can guide others toward life-changing discoveries.

It costs nothing and takes just a minute, but your words could be the spark that changes someone's journey. Simply scan the QR code or visit:

https://review.autoimmunityunlocked.org

Thank you for lending your voice to this project,

Anar R. Guliyev, M.D.
    Author

CONCLUSION

As I write this book, new research continues to reveal fascinating connections. I've learned that Alzheimer's disease appears to involve an autoimmune mechanism and that there is a link between Parkinson's disease and the body's microbiome. It's mind-boggling how much human beings rely on certain bacteria to ensure health and well-being.

A gut-brain connection might seem like science fiction. After all, they're completely separate organs. But the results of ongoing studies show that the tiny organisms living within us can, and do, affect many areas of the body, including the brain. This should come as no surprise, considering the immune system operates in every human organ and system.

It is alarming how many people are at risk of diseases related to immunity and the microbiome. Around 6% of the population has a diagnosed autoimmune disease, and another 6% will develop one in their lifetime. 30% of the population suffers from allergies, and 20% have food intolerances. Then, there's the increased risk of all kinds of cancer in people with compromised immunity. That's why I believe the 5R+ System is relevant for everyone—it targets common problems that underscore a multitude of health issues.

This begs the question: What are we doing to our bodies? In many ways, we treat them as poorly as the land we live on. Mankind has a bad reputation for replacing pristine forests and meadows with cities and monoculture farms. Industrialized modern living has wiped out much of the natural flora and fauna and created an environment that favors only a few pests that have adapted to life in our yards and wastelands. We continue to replace lush, robust ecosystems with a few fragile crops that constantly teeter on the edge of failure without our intervention—pesticides and chemical fertilizers. Our pets, whose ancestors navigated vast pastures and hunting grounds, now lose their way in their own neighborhood. They have lost their ability to survive in the wild.

A similar process is happening inside the human body. Our once robust and diverse microbiome is now fragile and lacking variety. Our immune cells are confused about who's friend or foe. And pathogens thrive on chronic inflammation.

 We don't just live in an ecosystem—we ARE an ecosystem, for and of the trillions of bacteria and immune cells that call our bodies home.

If you want to enjoy good health, these residents must be healthy too. And that means changing their entire ecosystem. It requires action on many fronts and adjustments to multiple factors.

The **5R+ System** is a structured roadmap that addresses these needs. Through significant changes to your diet and your internal and external environments, you can **RESTORE** your immune system and tame the autoimmunity beast. This is achieved by **REPOPULATING** your microbiome with healthy bacteria, **REDUCING** chronic inflammation, **REPAIRING** your intestinal epithelium, **REAWAKENING** your intestinal motility, and **RECONDITIONING** other factors beyond the digestive system.

My journey, and that of many others, is proof that the time, commitment, and effort it takes to stay on this path to healing is worth it. The effort you put into changing your lifestyle now enables you to live the life of your dreams—pain-free and full of vitality.

Research on the topics of autoimmunity and the microbiome is ongoing. Given time, we'll learn even more about the interconnection of these two fascinating topics, leading to a greater understanding and enhanced treatment strategies.

I am grateful to God for leading me in my research during the early 2000s on the link between autoimmune disease, the gut microbiome, and lifestyle. My healing was a miracle, but the miracle came in the form of understanding—a gift that can be shared with others. May this experience now help you in your journey to robust health.

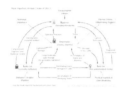

APPENDICES

APPENDIX 1. ILLUSTRATIONS, TABLES, AND VIDEOS

Scan the QR code to access the materials online.

https://book.
autoimmunityunlocked.
org/a1

———

APPENDIX 2. REFERENCES AND ADDITIONAL READING

Scan the QR code to access references, additional reading, and scientific publications online.

https://book.
autoimmunityunlocked.
org/a2

BONUSES

Scan the QR code to access additional materials online.

https://bonus.autoimmunityunlocked.org

BONUS 1. PRINTABLE MIND MAP OF 5R+ KEYS AND TACTICS

BONUS 2. THE ART OF FERMENTATION: DELICIOUS VEGETABLE AND DAIRY PROBIOTICS RECIPES

BONUS 3. FOOD BASKETS: FOODS RANKED BY THEIR IMPACT ON THE GUT-MICROBIOME-IMMUNE ECOSYSTEM

Made in United States
Cleveland, OH
19 June 2025

17838452R00216